TODAY, MOST CHILDLESS COUPLES *CAN* HAVE THE BABY THEY WANT.

Dr. Sherwin A. Kaufman—one of the nation's most respected specialists in the field of infertility—now presents the most up-to-date recent information and medical guidance:

- Where to get help when you need it
- The "fertility pill" and Pergonal
- Effects of abortion, the pill and IUD on fertility
- Causes of miscarriage
- Alternatives for the infertile, including artificial insemination
- Why infertility is on the rise
- How to increase your own chances for having a baby
- New techniques in treating infertility, from microsurgery to test tube births

"EXCELLENT"—*Woman's Day*

D1460871

BETTER HOMES AND GARDENS ® BABY BOOK

CHILDBIRTH AT HOME by Marion Sousa

CHOICES IN CHILDBIRTH by Dr. Silvia Feldman

COMPLETE BOOK OF BREASTFEEDING
by Marvin Eiger, M.D. and Sally Olds

THE FIRST TWELVE MONTHS OF LIFE
edited by Frank Caplan

IMMACULATE DECEPTION by Suzanne Arms

MOVING THROUGH PREGNANCY
by Elisabeth Bing

NAME YOUR BABY by Laureina Rule

NINE MONTHS READING: A MEDICAL GUIDE
FOR PREGNANT WOMEN
by Robert E. Hall, M.D.

PREGNANCY NOTEBOOK by Marcia Colman Morton

PREPARING FOR PARENTHOOD by Dr. Lee Salk

THE SECOND TWELVE MONTHS OF LIFE
by Frank and Theresa Caplan

SIX PRACTICAL LESSONS FOR AN EASIER
CHILDBIRTH by Elisabeth Bing

UNDERSTANDING PREGNANCY AND
CHILDBIRTH by Sheldon H. Cherry, M.D.

YOU *CAN* HAVE A BABY
by Sherwin A. Kaufman, M.D.

You *Can* Have A Baby

SHERWIN A. KAUFMAN, M.D.

**NEW HOPE FOR THE
CHILDLESS, INCLUDING THE
FACTS ABOUT TEST TUBE BIRTHS
& OTHER TECHNIQUES**

*This low-priced Bantam Book
has been completely reset in a type face
designed for easy reading, and was printed
from new plates. It contains the complete
text of the original hard-cover edition.*
NOT ONE WORD HAS BEEN OMITTED.

YOU CAN HAVE A BABY
*A Bantam Book / published by arrangement with
Elsevier/Nelson Books*

PRINTING HISTORY
*Elsevier/Nelson edition published November 1978
2nd printing . . . February 1980*
Bantam edition / May 1980

ISBN 0-553-13112-5

Published simultaneously in the United States and Canada

Bantam Books are published by Bantam Books, Inc. Its trademark, consisting of the words "Bantam Books" and the por-
trayal of a bantam, is Registered in U.S. Patent and Trademark
Office and in other countries. Marca Registrada. Bantam
Books, Inc., 666 Fifth Avenue, New York, New York 10019.

PRINTED IN THE UNITED STATES OF AMERICA

0 9 8 7 6 5 4 3 2 1

*To those I love—my wife, Claire,
and my sons, Kenneth, Keith, and Michael*

CONTENTS

PART THREE
AFTER THE TESTS: REAPPRAISAL

PART FOUR
SEX AND THE BIOLOGY
OF REPRODUCTION

TO THE READER

The purpose of this book is to survey the causes and treatment of infertility for those who need help.

Couples who have been unsuccessfully trying to have a baby tend to despair very quickly. They may be pleasantly surprised to learn in this book that they need not be so pessimistic. New medical advances have brought hope to the childless, more hope than in any previous generation.

But many couples are not aware of the help that is available, or else may be laboring under common myths and mistaken notions. Such couples are understandably frustrated, perhaps even bewildered. They would like to know what is wrong, and how they can be helped to have the child that would represent the fulfillment of their marriage, a product of their love. They, too, want to share the miracle that is the sight of a newborn baby and the knowledge that they have created it.

The field of infertility is unique and unlike any other medical specialty. It is the only known medical condition that concerns more than one person. It is also the only one in which the doctor starts out with two people and hopes to end up with three or more! It is surely the most personal branch of medical practice, dealing as it does with *the very essence of maleness and femaleness, and with sexuality. Management of infertility, therefore, requires the keenest insights, the greatest tact, the greatest compassion.*

—SHERWIN A. KAUFMAN, M.D.

YOU *CAN*
HAVE A BABY

Part One

THE BACKGROUND

1

HISTORICAL BACKGROUND

Sterility has been a human problem from the dawn of antiquity. In earliest times the woman who failed to conceive was looked upon as being cursed. Each culture had its own methods of dealing with the relief of infertility.

In ancient times astrology was used to map out the days or months best suited for fertility. Numerologists were also consulted, and were particularly busy figuring out the relationship between libido and phases of the moon which were believed to influence fertility.

The ancient Hindus worshiped both phallic symbols and figures of female genitalia. A hole in a tree or rock symbolized the female birth passage, and it was believed that women who passed through such a cleft would have improved fertility. The same custom is still followed in many lands retaining primitive rites.

The old wives' tale that an eighth-month baby will not fare as well as a seventh-month infant originated from ancient Hindu writings describing how in the eighth month a "vital force" was withdrawn from the child to the mother.

It was ancient Greece that gave us the father of medicine, Hippocrates, who was born in 460 B.C. Hippocrates observed that "serving wenches" exemplify women of unusually good fertility: "No sooner do they have intercourse with a man than they become pregnant on account of their sturdy physique and their leanness of flesh."

For the most part, however, fertility in ancient Greece was believed to be a favor from the gods, who had their own problems. One of the ancient Greek goddesses, Actemia, was so agonized at her own birth that she obtained from Zeus the gift of eternal virginity. Apparently she later changed her mind, for mythology records that she seduced young Endymion and subsequently had many children.

Because many regarded the breast as the seat of fertility, an obvious result was the multibreasted goddess. The celestial midwife, Artemis (Apollo's twin), is represented in one statue as having no fewer than sixteen well-formed breasts.

The Romans borrowed most of their medicine from Greece but later became engulfed in an era of decadence, promiscuity and prostitution, at which time medicine sank to a low level.

The Roman ruler Numa Pompilius decreed that if any woman died while pregnant the baby was to be cut from her abdomen without delay. This later became part of the Lex Caesare and probably represents the true derivation of "Caesarean section" (Caesar himself had a normal birth).

The Roman physician Soranus (second century A.D.) was probably the first "specialist" in obstetrics and gynecology, and his text on the diseases of women remains a classic. Included are signs by which we may know whether a woman if fertile:

"Those who are beyond the fourteenth or fifteenth year of age, not too long nor too thick set, not too fat, not too flabby, not too moist or too dry, with cervices not too open nor too closed, those who menstruate regularly—these are fertile. Those who do not possess large and fleshly loins and are mannish in their physique are sterile. Sterile also are those who are not shaped like a normal woman, too thin or too fat, too young or too old."

Soranus was not only interested in sterility, but was also the first to consider the plight of the infertile with special concern. He had a good knowledge of female anatomy and was the first to use a vaginal speculum to view the cervix. He thought that the most favorable time for conception was shortly after a menstrual period, and taught that staying in bed after intercourse may improve fertility.

Medicine remained at a more or less dormant level for many centuries thereafter. Sterility in the eighteenth century was treated empirically. In 1709, Carlo Musitano recommended obscene entertainment, still adhering to the belief that sexual gratification was essential for conception.

The relationship between infertility and ectopic (tubal) pregnancy was first suggested by Boehmer in 1752. It was thought to happen during the act of extramarital intercourse (illicit sex, discovered), resulting in the egg's failing to progress along the tube.

Actually it was not until 1786 that Spallanzani showed spermatozoa to be essential for fertilization, and not until 1827 that Van Kolliker demonstrated the origin of sperm and their fertilization of the ovum. It remained for Von Baer in the same year to discover the mammalian ovum.

James Marion Sims, one of the most famous of

early American gynecologists, wrote the classic *Clinical Notes on Uterine Surgery* in 1866. He was much interested in infertility problems, and in 1868 addressed the New York County Medical Society "On the Microscope as an Aid in the Diagnosis and Treatment of Sterility." His insistence on semen studies caused some strong reaction in the *Medical Times and Gazette*, which charged that "This dabbling in the vagina with speculum and syringe is incompatible with decency and self-respect."

In many lands today ancient customs are still adhered to. Hungarian peasant women bite their own afterbirths to ensure continued fertility in the future. Chinese and Javanese women actually eat some of the placenta to improve fertility.

It is a wise man who refrains from being too harsh upon or critical of ancient customs and folklore. I recall, many years ago, being impressed by the strange case of a woman who was operated on by a highly skilled gynecological surgeon. Two days later she had to be taken to the operating room again because of unexpected bleeding from the operative site. On close inspection, however, nothing unusual was seen; the bleeding had suddenly ceased. A few days later the same thing happened. After the third or fourth such episode the patient called aside the perplexed surgeon and related her suspicions—that she was under a "hex" and someone was sticking pins into her effigy. She thought she knew who it was and said that person would have to be stopped in order to break the spell. Because of the most unusual nature of the case the surgeon felt he had little to lose by bowing to superstition. A messenger was dispatched to the named individual. The pin-sticking ceased, and so did the bleeding.

In the words of Hippocrates, "Life is short, the art long, timing is exact, experience treacherous, judgment difficult."

2

GENERAL FACTORS
INFLUENCING FERTILITY

The ability to have children cannot be predicted from external appearances. Beauty and body build are no sure indicators of fertility. A healthy, virile-looking man is not necessarily more fertile than his scrawnier neighbor (look around you). Nor is the voluptuous woman always at an advantage when it comes to bearing children.

When pregnancy occurs easily, no thought is given to the complex mechanism involved. It just "happens." Only when the mechanism fails is any thought given to its many intricacies.

Every man and woman has a certain fertility potential—difficult to assess, but let's say good, fair, or poor. Pregnancy is always the result of the combined fertility of husband and wife. For example, a highly fertile man may have no difficulty impregnating his wife of relatively low fertility. On the other hand, if this man's own fertility were lower than average, or even average, a barren marriage might result. Similarly, a highly fertile woman may compensate for her husband's lesser potential.

The general health of the couple is of importance: a person who is run down, anemic, or otherwise in poor health is probably not functioning at optimum capacity.

FERTILITY AND AGE

For a woman there is also a definite relationship between fertility and age. Fertility begins in the teens. The first year or two that a young girl menstruates is usually without egg production, hence without fertility. (However, there are indeed numerous exceptions.) More commonly, fertility becomes established one to three years after the onset of menses, about the time the periods assume a regular pattern.

Thereafter fertility potential rises, reaching its optimum during a woman's twenties. During her thirties, there is a general reduction in a woman's fertility. The exact level of *individual* fertility at a given age cannot be stated precisely, since it depends upon previous potential. For example, a woman who at thirty had unusually good fertility is not likely to "drop off" significantly at thirty-five; whereas one who was borderline in fertility at thirty is very likely to be sub-fertile a few years later.

Age, as it relates to fertility, is the one factor over which neither doctor nor patient has any control, nor is there any way to reverse it. Therefore, from the practical point of view, a couple seeking help because of childlessness should do so sooner if the wife is in her thirties than if she is younger.

Then there is the question of fertility in women

after forty, and the relationship between fertility and menopause. By definition fertility comes to an end with menopause—or does it? Apparently not always, since the so-called "menopause baby" is a well-known entity. When the family is complete, such an event is usually greeted with dread, though sometimes with amusement, as in the play *Never Too Late*, which describes the incongruity of the unexpected mixed blessing.

Actually, pregnancy after menopause is rare. In fact, pregnancy during the late forties is sufficiently uncommon to have occasioned a number of surveys along this line. The consensus is that the chance of pregnancy after fifty is negligible.

Nevertheless, medico-legal opinions tend to play it safe. For example, the British courts concluded: "We cannot pretend to fix the age at which pregnancy ceases to be possible and beyond which it cannot occur." The common law in the United States concurs—that is, a woman "is conclusively presumed to be capable of bearing children until death."

Actually, a woman's fertility falls off with advancing age at about the same rate at which her eggs disappear from her ovaries. Physiologically speaking, then, a woman's fertility declines rapidly between forty and forty-five, and precipitously between forty-five and fifty, reaching near zero at fifty. This does not mean that women in their early forties should never seek help for infertility, since there may be some relatively simple, correctable impediment quite apart from age. It does mean, however, that no complicated procedure (such as tubal surgery or removal of small fibroids) would be undertaken in the face of the markedly diminished fertility due to age.

Regardless of exact age, once menopause is

reached there is no point in pursuing an infertility problem. Menopause, the physiological cessation of menses, indicates the loss of reproductive function.

How about the fertility of men as they grow older? Sperm studies of young and middle-aged men have shown there is no correlation between any aspect of the semen analysis and age. As the man passes from middle to old age there may be some decrease in sperm production, but apparently not enough to interfere with fertility. In fact, sperm motility remains undiminished in old age as long as *frequency* of intercourse is not greatly reduced.

So, while reproductive function in women ends with menopause, men can reproduce even into old age. There are reliable reports of men becoming fathers in their seventies, eighties, and even nineties.

BASIC PREREQUISITES FOR CONCEPTION

From the standpoint of reproductive anatomy and physiology, women are much more complicated than men. Unlike a man's reproductive organs, those of the female are well hidden and there are so many "parts" that much more can go wrong with a woman than with a man.

Impregnation *could* take place as early as a half hour after intercourse—about as long as it would take fast sperm to travel the few inches necessary to reach a waiting egg. But from the standpoint of probabilities, it is not that simple. In fact, any interruption in the necessary chain of events will impede or prevent conception, and when you stop to consider all the possible interruptions, you begin to wonder how *any* woman ever gets pregnant.

The basic prerequisites read almost like soap-opera cliffhangers: Will the sperm get into the cervix and into the womb? Will the egg be released from an ovary and enter the tube? Will they unite? Will the fertilized ovum be properly implanted in an adequately prepared uterus?

FAILURE TO CONCEIVE

In order to understand the various diagnostic procedures and treatments, one must first understand the various causes of failure to conceive. These might come under one of four headings: anatomical, physiological, associated with some physical disorder, or psychological.

ANATOMICAL CAUSES

There are very few anatomical causes for female infertility. Obviously the woman must have the necessary reproductive organs: a vagina, a uterus, tubes and ovaries. Congenital absence of any of these structures is exceedingly rare.

Some women wonder if their vagina is too short, complaining that seminal fluid flows out after intercourse. Actually, the vagina is a very elastic organ and accommodates itself to the penis very nicely. As far as semen running out is concerned, this is not unusual or abnormal, particularly if the volume of semen is high. Some semen almost always remains inside, near the opening to the womb, and this is the part that counts. Of course if a woman jumps up immediately after intercourse, to wash or dry herself, a good deal more semen will emerge than would otherwise be the case. This is not a good plan if the woman is trying to conceive. Some of my patients have even admitted douching immediately after intercourse, not realizing that this might hinder conception.

Unfortunately many women are told they have an immature or infantile (underdeveloped) womb and that because of this they will never be able to have a child. I say unfortunately, because this is the type of diagnosis that should not be made without the most careful evidence. What happens in many cases is that the uterus is sharply angulated upon itself and *feels* much smaller than it actually is. The doctor may easily mistake this for an underdeveloped uterus and hence err in his diagnosis. There is a simple way of measuring the uterus directly and thus avoiding this pitfall. In point of fact, even if the uterus does measure smaller than normal, it doesn't mean that pregnancy is not possible; I have lost count of the number of women with such a condition who have subsequently conceived.

Probably the most maligned diagnosis in gynecology is the so-called tipped or retroverted womb. By this is meant a uterus that is bent backward toward the rectum. I know of many women who have been told that they have a tipped womb, and that this will make conception difficult. Not so.

In the first place, a tipped uterus is very common. In many instances the uterus is actually so mobile that it may be tipped backward during one examination and tipped forward at another. This explains how two doctors can differ in their comments about its position. More important, however, the uterus that is tipped backward is not likely to be the cause of infertility as long as it is *movable*. The only exception occurs when a tipped uterus is combined with a semen volume which is consistently very low, making an insufficient "pool" to bathe the cervix.

However, if a tipped uterus is "fixed" in that position, this may have a definite relationship with infertility—not because of the position, but rather because of the underlying disorder causing the fixation.

PHYSIOLOGICAL CAUSES

Physiological causes of infertility have to do mainly with ovulation and the hormonal changes associated with it. Obviously if there is no egg there can be no pregnancy. Women who consistently fail to pass an egg usually do not menstruate either. However, just knowing that a woman menstruates does not mean that she necessarily ovulates.

In addition, there can be faulty ovulation, that is, eggs that are not as fertile as they might be, or else eggs that are passed sporadically, at very wide intervals.

PHYSICAL DISORDERS

An important category of infertility causes includes those associated with a specific physical disorder.

One of the most common of these is uterine fibroids. These are benign tumors; fibro-muscular growths that arise in the wall of the womb and may either grow outward, causing bumps on the surface, or inward, impinging on the lining of the womb. The exact cause of fibroids is unknown, but they seem to be associated with a greater-than-average level of estrogen production in the body. Many women with fibroids are able to conceive and have babies with no difficulty, particularly if the fibroids are small. However, if they should be located in such a way as to impinge upon the tubes in any way, they can be a cause of infertility. Furthermore, fibroids that are located mainly on the inside of the womb (submucous variety) can interfere with the embedding of a fertilized ovum.

Another physical disorder that may affect fertility is called "pelvic inflammatory disease." Most often this means an inflammation of the tubes that leaves them scarred and often crippled. The most common causes of such tubal inflammation are gonorrhea or infection following an unclean abortion. Other causes of tubal inflammation, such as tuberculosis, are seen more commonly in foreign countries. The tubes can also become inflamed as a result of an infection of a nearby organ such as a ruptured appendix. Even normal childbirth can produce an inflammatory reaction of the tubes, but in this latter instance, the inflammation is usually very low grade and not at all comparable in seriousness to the others mentioned. Anatomically speaking, the net effect of these infections is to close off or clog the tubes, sometimes with the destruction of the tubal lining.

Another physical disorder commonly associated with infertility is known as endometriosis. This is a condition in which bits of uterine lining are found *outside* the uterus—on the ovaries, tubes, intestines, etc. Since such tissue originates from the womb lining, it responds hormonally by "bleeding" each month. This can cause internal pain, experienced as very painful periods and other pelvic discomforts. However, more important from the standpoint of infertility, such internal droplets of blood set up a reaction that can cause scarring and narrowing of the tubes.

In about one third of the women with endometriosis, infertility is the primary complaint. Paradoxically, the failure to have children favors the spread of endometriosis. (This is often mentioned as a reason for a woman to have children while she is young.) Endometriosis is fairly common, but the cause is unknown.

Sometimes local physical disorders can interfere with fertility. For example, there may be a polyp (a small fleshy growth) at the entrance of the womb, or a cervical erosion (local infection) which interferes with sperm ascent.

PSYCHOLOGICAL CAUSES

The fourth but relatively uncommon cause for female infertility is that of psychological factors.

In my opinion, emotional frustration is more frequently the *result,* not the cause, of infertility. And it is incumbent upon the physician to make sure that no physical cause is overlooked before making that diagnosis.

On the other hand, every physician has encountered problems which are clearly psychologically caused.

For example, the fear of childbirth often results from something that the patient was told or overheard during an impressionable early age. Several patients in my own practice have told me that their mothers impressed them with the fact that they had "almost died" while giving them birth. Since daughters tend to identify with their mothers, it is not difficult to foresee the development of conflicts about pregnancy and childbirth.

There are other indirect, subtle ways in which the emotions can play havoc with physiological functions and cause infertility. One, for instance, is the emotional effect upon ovulation, the passage of an egg. If there is no ovulation, there can be no pregnancy. This lack can be a protective mechanism. As a matter of fact, an emotional cause should always be suspected whenever a woman with previously regular periods ceases to ovulate.

Another is the development of irregular staining that often accompanies lack of ovulation. This alone can effectively prevent intercourse ("How can I, when I'm bleeding all the time?"), thus limiting the chance of pregnancy, should ovulation unexpectedly occur. The emotional undertones are varied. The woman may simply be emotionally unprepared for the baby her husband is so eager for, and this is the way her body expresses its reluctance. Or there may be a marital problem serious enough to make the wife hesitant about becoming pregnant even though they may have decided to "save" the marriage by having a child.

Another way in which pregnancy can be prevented is by the psychological avoidance of intercourse due to pain. The woman develops an actual spasm of the vaginal muscles (known as vaginismus) which makes it impossible for the husband to "enter" sexually. This condition is usually present at the start of the marriage, and therefore comes to the physician's attention relatively early. It is surprising that such couples often come to the doctor with only the complaint of childlessness when the infertility problem is really secondary to the sexual one, which is, of course, disruptive to the relationship. Yet the supposed reason for the visit is nevertheless helpful in providing a clue to the probable underlying fear.

Vaginismus can also be caused by physical factors. These include common vaginal infections which produce discharge, itching, and irritation, and the treatment is of course directed toward the

17

specific disorder. Once the discomfort is eliminated the woman can again "relax," and the vaginal spasm vanishes.

Emotional vaginismus is much more complex. In many cases, the perceptive physician who is aware of the underlying involuntary spastic mechanism can then teach the patient to understand and overcome it. In other cases, the underlying problems are so deep-rooted that psychotherapy is advisable.

The inability to perform sexually is not confined to the female. Actually, it is more commonly a male problem. Thus, impotence and premature ejaculation are well-known sexual disturbances of emotional origin, and can also be responsible for infertility (see Chapter 6).

Of course, here I am discussing hesitancies about parenthood and fears of childbirth which are extremely strong and for the most part subconscious. I do not wish to imply that women who harbor mild fears are abnormal. On the contrary, *all* women have some anxiety about pregnancy and childbirth. This is perfectly natural. On the surface the woman may only express qualms about the discomforts of labor, but there are also much deeper anxieties—a fear of death, or that the baby will be stillborn, or even worse, deformed.

It is well to discuss such anxieties and bring them into the open, to prevent them from becoming suppressed or sufficiently strong to cause psychological infertility.

INDUCED ABORTION

Hospital wards throughout the country used to be filled with patients who developed infection of the tubes following self-induced or "illegal" abortion. Even after such infection was cleared up, the tubes were often left crippled. Two possible consequences of such inflammation are sterility or tubal pregnancy.

This is not meant as an indictment of abortion when a woman cannot physically or emotionally face the prospect of an unwanted pregnancy, but rather of the type of abortion that was so frequently done in a back-room office, ineptly or under unsterile conditions. The burden of compulsory pregnancy has been largely lifted by the legalization of abortion as a woman's right, so that the procedure can be done cleanly and efficiently, minimizing the chances of future sterility. However, even legal abortion can affect future fertility and is *not* advisable as a form of birth control (prevention is best).

CONTRACEPTION

It also seems obvious that the need for any kind of abortion is minimized by good contraceptive precautions regularly used. Contraception, then, is the first line of defense. More effective birth-control measures mean fewer abortions and their consequences. In other words, contraception does more than just prevent unwanted pregnancies. It can be a prime protector of future fertility.

THE PILL AND ITS EFFECT ON FERTILITY

Undoubtedly, the doctor will also question the couple about previous birth-control measures. Here the main interest surrounds the use or misuse of birth-control pills. Many women have the mistaken notion that upon discontinuing birth-control pills they will be "super-fertile," or that they will have a greater chance of multiple pregnancy. Neither statement is true. On the contrary, in some women, normal menstrual periods fail to resume upon discontinuing the pill, and this of course means lessened fertility.

It isn't that the pill is responsible for this condition (though sometimes it is). In most cases, the groundwork has already been laid prior to starting oral contraceptives. That is, the woman gives a history of having had menstrual irregularities *prior* to beginning the pills.

While contraceptive pills have been a great boon to millions, they must not be prescribed indiscriminately. There are some women for whom the pill is not the wisest choice. For example, if a young woman gives a history of grossly irregular cycles—skipping and the like—I am reluctant to prescribe oral contraceptives. The reason for this is that irregular cycles at best mean irregular ovulation; at worst, no ovulation at all. In short, the woman probably has reduced fertility already.

Of course, a young woman with irregular periods has no intention of testing her fertility at the time she requests the pill. But some time in the future she may want to have children. If she takes birth-control pills for several years, she will be *masking* the irregularity of her natural cycles, since the pills cause artificial bleeding on schedule. Thus, if her own cycles are destined to dwindle to none at all, she would be unaware of this while taking the pill. She may then be surprised to find, some years later when she is ready for children, that she has no spontaneous periods, a fact which would have been important to know in advance of her readiness for parenthood. Therefore, purely from the standpoint of fertility, I am opposed to the use of the pill to "regulate" widely spaced periods in younger women who have not completed their families. Some other method of contraception would be preferable.

There are also some women whose periods, though regular to begin with, fail to return upon discontinuation of birth-control pills. The proper choice of pill is important in minimizing this tendency. Fortunately, menstrual periods generally return spontaneously or with the help of special fertility drugs.

"LONG-LASTING" INJECTIONS

Periods more commonly fail to return for prolonged lengths of time following the discontinuation of "long-lasting" injections for contraceptive purposes. These injections usually consist of a progesterone-like compound which acts to prevent periods altogether for a specific length of time (one to six months). However, continued absence of menstruation for more than a year has been reported following discontinuation of the medication. It would therefore seem unwise to use this method of birth control for young women who have had no children.

THE INTRAUTERINE DEVICE

In the vast majority, fertility after discontinuation of the intrauterine device (IUD) seems to be essentially the same as before insertion, according to broad statistical evidence (barring a significant increase in the woman's age upon removal).

However, there is also evidence implicating the IUD in cases of low-grade (sometimes severe) pelvic inflammation, with the possibility of tubal scarring and infertility. Although the percentage is small, particularly when the physician avoids the IUD in any patient with a history suggestive of any previous pelvic infection, it should be kept in mind when a contraceptive choice is being made.

3

WHEN INFERTILITY
SHOULD BE SUSPECTED

A husband and wife decide to have a baby and abandon contraception. The next few months are then watched with keen anticipation. If the wife misses a period, well and good. However, if she does not miss her period, there is a bit more uneasiness with each passing month. After a few months this uneasy feeling gives way to anxiety and the suspicion that something is wrong. They begin to wonder if they will ever have a baby of their own. "What's wrong?" "When should we seek help?" "Where?" These are the inevitable questions that begin to arise even during the early months of trying to conceive, and come to the fore strongly when such trial appears to be prolonged.

Some women seek help for "sterility" after only two or three months. They are usually in a highly nervous state and cannot understand why they have not become pregnant after trying so hard. It is not generally known that despite boasts of conception after "one shot" it takes the average couple four to six months to achieve pregnancy. One reason for this is that the fertility of a woman's ovum varies from month to month. Incidentally, the term "sterility," although synonymous with "infertility," is rarely used because of its pessimistic implications.

In general, the young couple should continue their attempts to conceive for about a year before seeking help. If the wife is in her thirties, the time might be shortened about six months, since, as we know, fertility in women begins to decline with advancing years.

WHOM TO CONSULT?

Now for the second question: to whom shall the couple go for help? More specifically, to whom should the wife go for help, for it is most often the woman who accepts the onus of responsibility and visits a physician first.

THE FAMILY DOCTOR

The family doctor is generally the first to be consulted. This is a good "screening" procedure, since the family doctor is in an excellent position to eliminate the more obvious causes of infertility, or to counsel couples who have been trying only a very short time to wait longer. In his history-taking, he may discover, for example, that the husband has a habit of taking prolonged hot baths at bedtime. This can effectively interfere with sperm production, and the discontinuance of such a habit may be all that is required to restore male fertility.

In examining the husband, he may find undescended testes or varicocele and refer the man for a urological opinion. In examining the wife, he would be the first to note unexpected virginity and would then counsel the couple in sex anatomy and physiology. The family doctor is also in a good position to do a thorough physical examination on both partners and discover the presence of such disorders as severe anemia, diabetes, etc.

There are also instances where pregnancy is medically contraindicated—perhaps a severe heart or kidney disorder—and it would be well to know this in advance of seeking more specific help for an infertility problem.

THE SPECIALIST

If there are no obvious causes for infertility, your family doctor will probably want to refer you to a specialist who has had particular training and experience.

Most infertility specialists are gynecologists who have a special interest in this field. Some are endocrinologists, and those dealing exclusively with male infertility are usually urologists.

Many infertility specialists belong to the American Fertility Society, and names of its members in your area can be obtained from the Society's secretary, 1608 Thirteenth Avenue South, Birmingham, Alabama 35205.

Sometimes teams of doctors practice as a group and can coordinate the efforts of various specialists under one roof. This is also true in some hospital settings, and it is helpful to know your doctor's hospital affiliation, and whether it has a good gynecological and maternity service.

For those who cannot afford a doctor in private practice, there are infertility clinics in most parts of the country. Many are affiliated with the Planned Parenthood Federation of America and can be located by writing to that organization at 810 Seventh Avenue, New York, New York 10019.

No matter how good the professional qualifications of the specialist consulted, he must above all be sensitive to the special needs of the childless couple. A history of infertility is a history in frustration. One does not have to share that experience in order to empathize. One has only to know the joys of parenthood to understand the anguish of those couples who yearn for a child of their own and are continuously disappointed. They do not come to a doctor because of disease, but to obtain something they do not have. There is no area in medicine more sensitive and delicate than the study of infertility. Therefore the choice of doctor is particularly important.

It is not uncommon for childless couples to go from doctor to doctor. Sometimes it is because the specialist consulted is not sympathetic enough to their problem. Sometimes it is because he is unable to find anything wrong. And sometimes the specialist himself will suggest they consult another after a reasonable trial period, perhaps to confirm his own diagnosis and opinions. This does not mean that the patient will have to undergo repetition of every test previously done by another doctor. However, a new consultant may provide a fresh viewpoint or suggest something that has not been done or even thought of previously. We shall see presently, in this book, how many different nooks and crannies there are to be explored. It is not surprising, therefore, that some may be overlooked in anything less than a very thorough and methodical infertility investigation.

There is growing evidence that *infertility is on the rise*. Several reasons account for this: an increase in the incidence of venereal disease, particularly gonorrhea, which can severely damage the reproduction tracts in both men and women; the use of birth-control pills, which occasionally leads to prolonged delay before ovulation resumes after the pill is stopped; abortion, which in a small number can produce pelvic inflammation or weakness in the cervix that can lead to miscarriage in future pregnancies; the use of the intrauterine device (IUD), which may increase the risk of pelvic infection; and the current trend to delay marriage and childbearing until an age when fertility (for the woman) is naturally lower.

4

LEARNING THE EXTENT
OF THE PROBLEM:
THE FIRST CONSULTATION

Let us picture a husband and wife in a specialist's consultation room. They are tense and upset. They've been trying to have a baby for almost a year. They have many questions: Is it hopeless? If not, what are our chances? How long will it take to find out? What needs to be done? Will it hurt?

The understanding physician will first put the couple at ease. He might explain that their plight is indeed urgent but not unusual. About one of every ten married couples in the United States find themselves among the frustrated ranks of the infertile. Another 15 percent of wives are able to conceive, and then miscarry. This means that about 25 percent of couples, one in four, run into a problem.

Are infertility problems usually hopeless? On the contrary, with today's new tests and treatments, there is more hope for the childless than ever before. Only a few decades ago, the chances of successfully helping a childless couple were only about 20 percent. Today, new medical advances have more than doubled that figure; between 50 and 70 percent of childless couples can be helped to have a baby.

In order to get as complete a picture as possible, the physician will ask certain questions. How long have you been trying to conceive? In general, the shorter the duration of infertility, the better the chances of having a baby. He will also ask the duration of marriage before attempted conception; here again, the shorter the "waiting" time, the better the overall prognosis. No doubt he will ask about menstrual periods in great detail (menstrual periods are really a history of ever-hopeful preparations for pregnancy).

During the course of history-taking the doctor will ask about average frequency of intercourse. The question has relevance only in relation to adequacy of exposure to pregnancy. Thus, if a couple reports a total frequency of two to three times a week, the exposure is, for all practical purposes, entirely adequate. Obviously if total frequency is far less, say once in three or four weeks, the chances of conception are correspondingly diminished, and there are instances where the *spontaneous* frequency of intercourse is so low that this may be a cause of infertility. In such couples it is necessary to explore the reasons for the lack of desire (or response). Here the unsatisfactory sexual relationship takes precedence over the infertility problem. Solving the former may well solve the latter.

Incredible as it may seem, every doctor has also had the experience of examining a woman who complains of infertility and finding that she is completely virginal, with an intact hymen—

indicating that the marriage has never been consummated.

In pursuing the medical history, the doctor will question the couple about past illnesses, particularly those which may have a direct bearing upon fertility. Probably the most devastating is venereal disease. The most common venereal disease is gonorrhea. Stated bluntly, gonorrhea can cause irreversible sterility in both sexes. In the male it does so by scarring the sperm-carrying ducts; in the female by destroying and scarring the delicate lining of the tubes—but only if the disease is permitted to get that far. This is why it is so urgent that symptoms of gonorrhea be reported and treated as soon as possible after exposure. Early symptoms in men may consist only of some burning on urination and/or a yellowish discharge from the penis. In *women* there may only be some vaginal discharge or urinary discharge and burning. In 80 percent there are *no* obvious symptoms.

A diagnosis of gonorrhea is best made by special cultures of the discharge, especially from the cervix, in women. During the early stage of the disease a cure is usually possible with antibiotics. However, once the disease has progressed up to the tubes (or testicles) it's another matter entirely. Even if treatment is begun shortly after this happens, some damage has already been done. If treated without further delay, fertility may still be salvaged. But often there is impairment of fertility leading either to difficulty in conceiving or to such complications as tubal pregnancy resulting from a fertilized egg's getting stuck in a damaged tubal lining.

In taking a medical history, the doctor will also want to know about previous pregnancies, miscarriages, or abortions, any of which may influence future fertility.

Often there are clues during history-taking that the emotional component has a significant bearing on the problem. For example, a doctor questioning a woman who consults him for infertility may ask her whether she has any difficulty reaching orgasm. This does not mean that orgasm is necessary for conception. Indeed, there is no evidence that it is. However, the question frequently provides the opportunity for the patient to go into a discussion of possibly important marital strife that she otherwise would have been hesitant to discuss. This in turn may lead to further questions regarding the possibility of emotional causes for the infertility problem.

I remember one woman who told me that she felt the need to get up to urinate immediately after intercourse. It made no difference whether she emptied her bladder just before intercourse; she still had this need directly afterward and always managed to have some urine to pass at that time. The amazing thing is that it did not occur to this couple that such a "ritual" made conception less likely. More important, the wife was unaware that there was any emotional need on her part to avoid getting pregnant, insisting that she craved a baby as soon as possible. It was only after a few psychotherapeutic sessions that she admitted her fears regarding pregnancy and childbirth. The infertility study was halted while she went into psychotherapy to gain a clearer understanding of her feelings.

One of the questions the physician is asked most frequently is, "Doctor, is it all in my head?" The public is well aware of the psychosomatic aspect of disease. In fact the diagnosis of "psychological infertility" arises inevitably whenever the couple suspects, or the doctor suggests, that there

31

is "nothing wrong." In those cases, it seems to me that there is an almost too eager tendency on the part of many infertile women to blame their plight on "nervousness." Are they not jittery? anxious? increasingly depressed? Of course they are. But are these symptoms the cause of their infertility, or the result? Any time a basic human impulse as strong as the maternal (or paternal) instinct is thwarted, nervousness is not an unnatural reaction. I believe that most such women are simply reacting to the frustration of infertility. Nor does preexisting nervousness exempt a woman from the added frustration of a barren marriage; her frustration then becomes even more acute.

Unfortunately, too many couples are told there is nothing wrong on the basis of incomplete testing.

The factors responsible for infertility can be few or many, obvious or obscure. Whether they are brought to light depends very much on the interest, skill and experience of the doctor taking the history and doing the necessary examinations. Even a simple question like "Have you had any operations?" and the equally simple answer, "Only an appendectomy many years ago," are of importance—but only if one is aware that acute appendicitis can produce scarring of the tubes and subsequent infertility.

At the same time, the physician sensitive to the needs of the childless couple is well aware that the successful outcome of an infertility study is not just the gathering of clues, or the opening up of previously closed tubes, or even the occurrence of pregnancy itself. *Successful outcome means the actual birth of a baby,* a baby that has been wanted very much for a very long time.

After history is taken and the initial physical examination completed, any obvious defects are corrected without delay. For example, if the woman has a polyp in the cervix, this is removed—usually a simple office procedure. Or if she has an erosion of the cervix, this is treated by cautery, another simple and quite painless office procedure.

Usually the situation is much more complex, and a detailed investigation is needed to uncover every possible cause of the couple's present infertility. Such a complete study is called a "work-up."

I want to say a word here regarding the common fear that infertility tests are very painful. This is highly exaggerated. While some of the tests can cause transient cramping, even this can be minimized by the judicious use of instruments and also by the injection of a local anesthetic near the uterus to promote relaxation and decrease discomfort.

The experienced physician will know without being asked that couples consulting him because of infertility will want to know, "Why are we unable to have a baby? What can you do to help us? How long will it take?" And knowing this, he answers the questions at once and outlines his plan for diagnosis.

The two outlines that follow—"The Essential Prerequisites for Conception" and "The Infertility Work-up"—are the core of this book, as they are of any infertility study.

5

THE ESSENTIAL PREREQUISITES FOR CONCEPTION AND THE INFERTILITY WORK-UP

In anticipation of the many questions that all couples will have when confronted with infertility, I like to begin by outlining the various steps necessary to unravel the "mystery"—steps which are as methodical as detective work.

These are the essential prerequisites for conception:

1. The husband must produce sperm of adequate quantity and quality.

2. The sperm must gain entry not only into the vagina but into the womb itself during the wife's fertile period.

3. The wife must ovulate (produce a mature ovum, or egg).

4. The egg must be of good quality.

5. The wife's tubes must be open to receive the egg each month and to permit the entry of sperm.

6. The tubes and womb must be unobstructed

to permit a fertilized egg free passageway into the uterus, which should also have a lining favorable for the embedding and growth of an embryo.

7. The various glands concerned with reproduction must be working harmoniously.

These are the conditions for conception for any couple.

Specific tests exist for each of these essentials. They are discussed in detail in subsequent chapters but may be outlined here as follows:

THE INFERTILITY WORK-UP

1. A semen analysis for sperm quality.

2. An after-intercourse test during the fertile period to see if the sperm have ascended into the uterus.

3. Basal temperature graphs to establish that ovulation is occurring.

4. An "egg test" (endometrial biopsy) to assess the quality of the ovum.

5. A tube test (gas insufflation—the Rubin test) to see if the tubes are freely open.

6. An x-ray of the uterus and tubes to reveal their inner outline.

7. Various blood and urine tests for the function of specific glands, such as the thyroid, adrenal, pituitary, and, of course, the ovaries. In this connection the study of cervical secretions may also be helpful. In addition, bacterial cultures and immunological tests may also be taken.

8. Endoscopy: direct visualization of the pelvic organs.

An infertility work-up can usually be completed within three to four months. This allows time to repeat any tests that showed abnormalities. Gradually the pieces of the jigsaw puzzle begin to form a picture. At the completion of the study, the doctor should, of course, have a conference with both the husband and wife to explain the results, as well as the recommended treatment.

Part Two

THE WORK-UP

6

MALE INFERTILITY AND
THE SPERM TEST

Time was when infertility was considered strictly a female problem. Men considered themselves absolved of any responsibility for barren marriages. Indeed it was the custom in many primitive cultures (a custom still retained in some lands) for the husband to divorce his wife if she bore him no children within a certain length of time. It apparently never dawned on the husband who had a succession of "sterile" wives that the problem might be his.

We know now that the male is fully responsible for infertility in about 20 percent of the cases, and partially responsible in about 20 percent more. He is thus either wholly or partly involved in 40 percent of all cases. It is no longer just the wife who comes for help.

The knowledge that husbands share responsibility in infertile marriages may make many men feel insecure. Men are just as sensitive about their fertility as women—perhaps even more so. Most men want to be fathers, and the inability to initi-

39

ate pregnancy strikes at their very manhood and virility.

THE SPERM

Exactly where does the "male seed" come from? The formation of sperm takes place in thin (seminiferous) tubules in the testicles. Other cells secrete the male hormone (testosterone), giving the man his "maleness." The pituitary gland influences the production of testosterone by a delicate system of checks and balances.

The testicles are located in the scrotum, which nature has wisely placed outside the body in order to keep it as cool as possible. Sperm are harmed by heat, and the location of the scrotum makes it four to five degrees cooler than body temperature. Men who take daily prolonged hot baths can unknowingly depress their sperm production, but this is reversible when the habit is stopped. Some men have been known to unwittingly depress their sperm by wearing tightfitting suspensories, which press the testicles too close to the warmth of the body. Fever can have the same effect, dropping the sperm count to near zero, with equally dramatic restoration a few weeks later. Men needn't worry about extreme external temperature changes as far as sperm are concerned. The temperature in the scrotum is automatically regulated by the dartos muscle, which pulls the scrotum up nearer to the body in cold weather and relaxes it in warm weather, as any man can testify.

Spermatozoa were actually unknown until about three hundred years ago. Anton van Leeuwenhoek, a Dutch dry-goods clerk, took up the hobby of grinding lenses back in the seventeenth century. His young assistant, Hamm, became curious about semen and was the first to discover sperm. Leeuwenhoek then described what he saw to the Royal Society of London with the comment, "And if your lordships should consider such matters either disgusting or likely to seem offensive to the learned, I earnestly beg that they be regarded as private and either be published or suppressed as your lordships' judgment dictates."

A spermatozoon has an oval head, short body and long tail. Sperm are produced in fantastic numbers; as many as a half billion may be ejaculated at one time. During his lifetime a human male may produce more than a trillion sperm.

The bulk of an ejaculation consists of secretions from the seminal vesicles and prostate gland. The seminal vesicles were wrongly named on the presumption that they stored sperm. The prostate gland is a three-lobed structure the size of a walnut, surrounding the upper part of the urethra, the tube leading into the bladder.

Considering that sperm were microscopically seen three hundred years ago, it seems incredible that evaluation of male infertility by semen analysis did not take place until fairly recently—in 1929.

A semen analysis is one of the first steps in any infertility investigation. This should be done only by one who is experienced in this particular field; many routine laboratories are not. As a rule the gynecologist or urologist specializing in infertility has a broader understanding of this subject and the importance of accuracy and correct interpretation.

WHAT IS "NORMAL"?

To understand what subnormal semen is, one must know the wide range of normality. This is not as easy as it sounds. More than thirty years ago I became interested in this subject and undertook to answer the question: What is a normal semen? in a study published in a medical journal in 1946. In this study I obtained sperm samples from men whose wives had had two or more children, no miscarriages, and *were pregnant at the time of the study*. The results showed the wide range of "normality," and also helped to topple some of the old standards that had remained on the books for years. This point is particularly important because there is a tendency on the basis of a sperm analysis to place a label on a man, such as "weak" or "low" or even "good," with only very sketchy data to support such an opinion. For one thing, no conclusions should be drawn on the basis of a single semen analysis. If it is poor in any way, the test should be repeated. There are too many extraneous reasons why a given specimen may be poor on any certain day, and unless there is a consistent pattern, the opinion should be held in abeyance.

I recall one husband who brought his semen sample to me for examination. From the past history I expected a normal specimen. When I saw how poor it actually was, I at first expected that he had lost some of it in collection or in transit but he assured me that he had not. I then questioned whether there was any moisture in the bottle, since water has a spermicidal effect. But the bottle was perfectly dry, he was quite certain. Well, it turned out that this man had had the flu about three weeks before. What I was seeing was still the effects of marked sperm depression that ordinary illness can cause. The examination of his specimen a few weeks later revealed a perfectly normal picture.

THE SEMEN ANALYSIS

Exactly what is a semen analysis? The husband is asked to submit his semen, either self-induced or after intercourse by withdrawing and ejaculating into a clean, dry glass jar. Care should be taken not to lose any of the specimen, especially the first portion, since it contains about three quarters of all sperm and also those of best quality.

No set number of days of abstinence is required before collection; it should simply be taken at the couple's usual interval of coital frequency, so that it is a representative sample. The specimen is then examined within 2–3 hours of collection for volume, count, motility, survival time, and anatomic types.

Ejaculate volume has little to do with fertility except in the extremes. If it is consistently too low (less than 1.0 cc, which is 15 drops), there may be too little of the seminal "pool" for conception. On the other hand, if the volume is very high (over 8.0 cc), it is associated with poor fertility for reasons that are often obscure.

The sperm count varies from day to day and from hour to hour. In general, it diminishes with frequent intercourse (e.g., daily) as does the volume produced. However, the motility of the sperm (the most important aspect) is unaffected by frequent intercourse; this plus the increased exposure offsets the lowered volume and count, up to a point.

I am always reminded of a couple in my practice who had intercourse "once or twice daily" for years. The sperm in this case were so depleted (but not the husband evidently) that the "cure" was simply to let up for a few days to permit some regeneration. I hasten to add that this type of problem is unusual. Frequent, even daily, coitus may have no significant effects on the sperm of a man whose semen quality is high to start with. On the contrary, sperm count can be depressed by long periods of abstinence, and the motility may also suffer. In general, *increased* (rather than decreased) frequency of coitus improves chances of conception at any level of fertility, probably because sperm motility is improved by more frequent ejaculation.

It used to be thought and taught that any count under sixty million (per cc) was subnormal and would lead to difficulty with conception. We know today that this is not true. For one thing, the number of sperm varies from day to day and should never be considered static. This does not mean that the man whose count is forty million (per cc) one day is likely to have one hundred and forty million the next, but it does mean that he should not be branded with one particular number as his. In fact, it is now generally recognized that any count above twenty million may fall into the broad category of normal, *provided that other features of the sperm are adequate*. However, an average sperm count among men of good fertility is around one hundred million per cc.

Perhaps the most important feature of a semen analysis is the number of *moving* sperm, especially the quality of motion. If semen is examined *immediately* after ejaculation, the motility of the sperm is characteristically "poor" for a while, since semen coagulates (gels) at first. It takes several minutes for semen to liquefy, and maximum motility is not reached until full liquefaction occurs. This time lag is a laboratory phenomenon;

in the body, sperm are actively motile *immediately* on gaining entrance into the cervix.

When sperm are examined after liquefaction, the percentage of motile sperm is noted as well as the quality of motion. Normally, more than 50 percent of the sperm should be moving (within two to three hours of ejaculation) and the quality of motion should be uniformly good. As the hours pass, the number of moving sperm gradually decreases, but even after twenty-four hours some sperm should still be moving.

Another interesting aspect of sperm is their structural shapes (morphology), as seen on a stained smear. There should normally be no more than 40 percent "abnormal" types. *All* men exhibit a certain number of "abnormally" structured sperm. This has nothing to do with abnormal offspring. The sperm morphology has a surprisingly constant pattern. In fact, some men may be identified by their sperm, as by fingerprints.

When the semen analysis is completed, an overall evaluation is made of the sperm quality in terms of fertility potential. Often more than one specimen is needed to arrive at a meaningful evaluation.

SPERM DEFICIENCY

When sperm deficiency is only moderate, general health is built up. Thyroid is given if a deficiency of this hormone has been demonstrated. A survey of the pituitary and adrenal gland function may also be undertaken. Some doctors have prescribed various doses of male hormone, and other hormonal preparations have been tried with varying degrees of improvement. The most dramatic results have been associated with correction of varicose veins of the scrotum (varicocele), which is discussed on p. 51.

WEAK SPERM

One of the most interesting and most successful methods of handling "weak" sperm is by means of the partitioned ejaculate, the first portion in one bottle, the remainder in another. If a drop from each bottle is examined under a microscope, it looks as though it were from two different men, so strikingly superior is the first portion as a rule. This principle is used therapeutically by placing the first portion of the ejaculate at the opening of the wife's womb at a time in her cycle when she is considered most fertile. Some doctors give the sperm an extra boost by inseminating the superior portion, collected in a sterile jar, almost into the cavity of the uterus by a special technique. These are "artificial insemination" procedures using the husband's semen, as distinguished from those using a donor's semen. When done for weak sperm, the success rate of artificial insemination with the *husband's* semen depends directly on the quality of sperm obtained by use of the partitioned ejaculate. In my experience, the pregnancy rate is improved when the sperm are given a higher boost.

A patient I'll call Marian consulted me for infertility about two years ago. A thorough investigation revealed no abnormalities except that her husband had a subnormal semen with generally poor motility. A partitioned ejaculate revealed the first portion to be good enough for therapeutic husband insemination. This superior portion was placed at the opening of the womb for three cycles at ovulation time without success. The fourth cycle I inseminated the first portion of semen almost into the uterine cavity. The wife became pregnant that month and was subsequently delivered of a normal girl. It is probable that if this couple decides to have another baby, the same procedure will have to be used.

In considering the treatment of infertile couples where the principal deficiency is "weak" sperm, one must not lose sight of the fact that anything that raises the wife's fertility potential will tend to compensate for lessened fertility on the husband's part. For example, a "fertility pill" formerly used for another purpose is now being used more generally in an effort to obtain *better*-than-average female fertility. In addition, certain hormonal products for the wife may also help to create a better environment for fertilization or implantation. Such multiple therapeutic measures have produced superior results in recent years in terms of successful pregnancies.

No man should be told that it is impossible for him to father a child, unless he has absolutely no sperm on successive examinations. Pregnancies have been known to occur with sperm counts as low as one million per cc.

FROZEN SPERM

A word about frozen sperm. Human sperm stored in liquid nitrogen at $-196°$ Centigrade have retained their motility and fertilizing capacity for more than four years, according to certain techniques reported. However, only sperm of good quality have been used successfully in this manner. Unfortunately, at the present time, freezing sperm of poor quality (or pooling such sperm before freezing) does not result in sperm of superior quality.

LACK OF SPERM

An entirely different problem obtains if the husband has no sperm at all or practically none. In the most severe cases, where there is very little or no sperm production, a biopsy (small slice for examination) of the testicle may be taken to distinguish between lack of production and blockage due to past disease. This is done by a urologist. Relief of blockage is occasionally attempted surgically; but there is no remedy for lack of production. The choices available to such a couple are discussed in Chapter 18.

IMPOTENCE

Male impotence is the inability to carry out the act of sexual intercourse. The man cannot maintain an erection, or, in rare cases, cannot ejaculate. In either case the wife cannot become pregnant, since no sperm are deposited in the vagina.

Like vaginismus in women, impotence is disruptive to a couple's sexual relationship, and as such is threatening to the marriage. Obviously a search for the cause takes first priority, and it usually requires a psychotherapeutic approach. Sometimes it is discovered that the basic problem is fear of causing pregnancy—either an anxiety that the wife will not survive it or an emotional unpreparedness for fatherhood. Once these problems are resolved (and this is not simple), impotence disappears and there may be no further barrier to fertility.

There are other instances, however, in which the husband is impotent and the wife has fully accepted this as a permanent way of life. The marriage seems quite durable and the couple seek help for their problem, which is infertility.

In cases of erectile impotence, insemination of the husband's self-induced specimen into the wife's vagina or cervix during her mid-cycle usually results in pregnancy within a short time provided there are no other impediments. The reason the success rate is so high is that there is nothing standing in the way of conception except the husband's impotence. Insemination with the husband's sperm hurdles that particular impediment.

In almost every such case I have treated, the husband was also going to a psychotherapist for help with his basic problem. Practically all cases of impotence are emotionally caused. In a few instances, impotence is a result of physical injury and paralysis, in which case the same insemination procedure is carried out.

Less frequently I have encountered husbands with ejaculatory impotence, the inability to discharge any sperm, there being no difficulty with maintaining an erection and otherwise performing sexually. Such situations are much more intriguing from the psychological point of view, as they seem to point directly at the subconscious need to avoid impregnation. If both psychotherapy and neurological investigation fail to change the status, the only solutions (other than remaining childless) are adoption or donor insemination.

I recall one couple who were seemingly happily married. They had a most satisfactory sex life in that the husband was able to maintain an erection for prolonged periods of time. However, at no time was he able to ejaculate. (This inability to discharge sperm went back to his adolescent years.) Both claimed a strong desire to have children.

Because of the husband's unusual disorder he had had prolonged psychotherapy prior to consulting me. His desire for children remained unshaken. If there was any reason why his subconscious did not want him to father children, it was not evident to his psychiatrist. Neurological consultation had also proved negative. They came for donor insemination and I agreed, with some hesitancy.

The wife became pregnant promptly. I watched the husband's reaction with particular interest. He was as happy and proud as any father could be. This was a number of years ago. They have since returned for another insemination, which was just as successful, and now consider their family complete. Interestingly, although his wife is willing to use contraception he remains unable to ejaculate even under the present circumstances.

OTHER CAUSES OF
MALE INFERTILITY

What can be done for the infertile male? Much depends on the specific nature of the deficiency as well as the physical examination. A careful history will often provide the clue. Perhaps there is a history of undescended testicles, or severe infections, or venereal disease. There may be a glandular deficiency such as thyroid. The use of certain toxic drugs, exposure to x-rays, poor nutrition, excessive use of alcohol—any of these may contribute.

As we saw earlier, the effect of gonorrhea upon fertility can be devastating. Infertility may also result from perfectly "respectable" diseases. One of the most common is mumps. Lucky is the boy who develops mumps as a child, rather than in later years. It is after puberty that mumps may attack the testicles (in 20 percent of cases), causing severe inflammation (orchitis) and usually complete sterility. All prepubescent males should be immunized against mumps to avoid testicular mumps in later life.

One should be wary of being dogmatic. I will not soon forget one husband who, after considerable treatment for subnormal sperm, was able to impregnate his wife no fewer than three times, with the result that they had three daughters to their credit. Some years later this man developed mumps with involvement of both testicles, and assumed afterward that he was sterile. The couple happily abandoned contraception—but to their surprise, there was apparently enough regeneration of his sperm to make him fertile again, and his wife conceived once more.

In recent years much attention has been directed toward the correction of varicose veins of the scrotum (varicocele). Such surgical correction by ligation has resulted in a significant number of pregnancies (if the wife is of normal fertility). The dominant therapeutic effect seems to be improvement in sperm motility, but it is not clear by what mechanism such benefit occurs. It is also paradoxical that the presence of varicocele need not be accompanied by any impairment of sperm quality. Although the causes and exact incidence of varicocele are debatable, there is no question but that it is a major cause of male infertility, and amenable to treatment in a high-enough percentage of cases to warrant thorough investigation.

7

THE AFTER-INTERCOURSE
TEST

Regardless of how fertile the sperm are, they must be able to reach the egg in order to fertilize. That means that they must first escape the normally hostile vaginal environment by entering the opening of the womb (cervix), then ascend through the cervical canal into the dark cavern of the womb itself. With no signposts to guide them, they must travel farther to enter the uterine opening of each tube. They must then travel against the current of the tubal lining to its outer portion where, hopefully, an ovum will be waiting or will soon arrive. Furthermore, about half the sperm, not knowing which tube will harbor the egg, unwittingly enter the wrong tube.

How is the physician to find out what is happening? He already has some idea of what the husband's sperm are like in the *bottle*. Now the question to be answered is, "What are the sperm like in the *body?*" The answer, or at least a partial answer, to this question is found in the after-intercourse test, also called the post-coital test, or Sims-Huhner test. This test offers microscopic evidence as to whether sperm have migrated freely through the cervical secretions into the uterine cavity.

The after-intercourse test was first described by J. Marion Sims over a hundred years ago, in 1869. A further report was given by his son, H. Marion Sims, in 1888. However, the test remained dormant for many years until popularized by another physician, Max Huhner, in 1913.

THE SIMS-HUHNER TEST

How is this test performed? Several hours after intercourse (there is no need to rush) secretions are taken from various levels of the cervical canal for microscopic examination; some doctors also take a sample from within the uterine cavity. The test is conducted in mid-cycle as close to ovulation as possible, since the cervical secretions are most hospitable to sperm at that time.

Normally, there should be large numbers of actively motile sperm throughout the cervical canal, moving without impediment in a background of clear, watery mucus. The best sperm reach the higher levels, becoming fewer in number as they ascend the reproductive tract. Samples of secretion taken directly from the inside of the womb show the fewest number of sperm, but all of excellent activity. They had to be to get there.

How do sperm get into the uterus? We know that sperm are capable of moving under their own power, as can be observed under the microscope. However, the speed with which they reach the upper portion of the reproductive tract has made many investigators wonder if there is perhaps another mechanism, such as contractions of the muscular walls of the uterus, which aids in transporting the sperm. There is no documented evidence that sperm move upward with deep inhalation or exhalation, or with orgasm.

Although the exact mechanism of sperm ascent remains obscure, it may nevertheless be said that, whatever the manner, sperm do make a *very* rapid ascent. This was shown by Sobrero and Mac-Leod, who did post-coital tests within one to one-and-a-half *minutes* after intercourse and found active sperm in the cervical canal. Another example of how sperm travel, even under great odds, was demonstrated in an experiment I conducted in 1951 wherein the sperm were able to *pass a spermicidal jelly barrier* in a matter of minutes and enter the cervix in a significant number of cases. Rapidity of sperm migration has been shown even more dramatically by Rubenstein and co-workers, who were able to recover sperm from the *fallopian tubes* during an operation performed within thirty minutes after coitus in patients who had been scheduled for surgery.

These data serve to explain graphically why it is that a douche taken after intercourse is an ineffective contraceptive. No woman can run fast enough.

What is the relationship between sperm migration and female orgasm? It used to be thought that orgasm aids in the ascent of sperm through some mechanical process, but this has never been observed. We know too that pregnancy takes place regularly in the absence of orgasm. Nor is the enjoyment of intercourse necessary for fertility. In 1886, J. Marion Sims conducted an experiment in which a man had intercourse with his wife while she was under general anesthesia. She became pregnant from this single coitus, "thus showing that mere sensual enjoyment in the female played no role." One could also observe that the subject was rather well relaxed.

It is astonishing to note the number of sperm ejaculated in comparison with the few that finally reach the egg. Most sperm die in the vagina, where they are initially deposited. In that hostile environment they can live for only one to three hours at the most, sometimes only for minutes. Some doctors have postulated that the normally acid secretion of the vagina is too detrimental to sperm, but other researchers have pointed out that sperm are just as short-lived in the vagina of a cow, which has an alkaline reaction. In any event, those sperm which do enter the cervix find themselves in a much more favorable environment. In fact, sperm can live very nicely in the cervix for at least forty-eight hours, and have been recovered from this area in some cases after several days. It is estimated that sperm have a similar longevity in the uterus and tubes—from two to several days, although there is some question about their fertilizing capacity after the first two or three days.

POOR RESULTS

What if no sperm are found in the tested secretions, or too few, or only inactive ones? This picture could result from inherently weak sperm—a condition which should be suspected from the examination of the fresh semen in the bottle. However, if the sperm are not inherently weak, the poor post-coital result could stem from hostile cervical secretions.

Unfavorable cervical secretions are found *normally* after ovulation has occurred, or if it is too many days before ovulation. However, if these are not the reasons, the fault may be within the cervix—for example, there may be various inflammatory conditions resulting in a thick, impenetrable mucus. The microscope or special cultures give the answer.

Suppose the infertility study shows that the woman has a chronic infection of the cervical canal which filters out the sperm and does not permit them to ascend into the uterus. In such situations, treatment is directed toward clearing up the chronic cervical infection by cauterization and sometimes antibiotics. In some cases, if this promises to take too long, the cervix can be bypassed by placing the husband's sperm through a thin tube directly up to the cavity of the womb. This is known as therapeutic husband insemination and requires a special technique.

Carol and Henry typify such a problem associated with infertility. Carol had a long-standing, non-irritating vaginal discharge. Examination revealed no abnormalities other than the cervical infection, which was also causing immobilization of sperm (proven on the post-coital test). After three months of treatment of her cervix, the discharge had finally ceased. However, pregnancy still did not take place, and the post-coital test still showed sperm immobilization. That is, the infection no longer produced external (overt) symptoms such as discharge, but the microscopic picture indicated that it would probably take a much longer time to clear up completely. In order to save time, I decided to bypass the cervical canal by instilling a portion of the husband's semen directly up to the uterine cavity. Carol became pregnant during the second cycle of treatment.

Sometimes cervical secretions are unfavorable not because of infection, but because of a hormonal imbalance. In such cases small doses of estrogen often improve the receptivity of the secretions through which the sperm must pass. When an unfavorable cervical secretion is the *only* factor inhibiting fertility, the prognosis for parenthood is generally favorable.

Another possible but much more obscure cause of a poor post-coital test is an immunological ("allergy") reaction, which is discussed on p. 116.

8

THE BASAL
TEMPERATURE GRAPH

In the field of infertility, the basal body temperature graph has been a boon or a bane, depending
on the use that has been made of it, by whom, and
for what purpose.

First of all, it is fascinating. It seems to satisfy
the gambling instincts of many women (will it go
up? down? stay the same?).

Men are envious. The basal body temperature
graph of a man is very uninteresting: it shows no
appreciable changes. Men are also angered by it. I
shudder to think of how often it has happened
that a man awakens in the morning and, still half
asleep, reaches out for his wife only to hear the
familiar: "Not until I take my temperature, and
then we'll see." The temperature graph has probably come closer to causing marital discord than
any single test ever devised, and the saddest part
is that it needn't do so at all.

WHAT IS IT?

About a hundred years ago, an English country gentleman by the name of Squire (*sic*) reported to his medical society that he had discovered a relationship between basal temperatures and ovulation. However, it was not until many decades later that anyone really demonstrated the usefulness of this relationship.

The procedure is as follows. A woman records her oral temperature each morning on awakening, having shaken down the thermometer the night before. That's all there is to it. If this is done from the start of one period to the next and the temperatures recorded on a graph, a line connecting them (as children connect animal pictures) will show a typical "biphasic" graph.

In a normal pattern the first phase usually shows temperatures below 98° F. and is under the dominance of estrogenic hormone. Somewhere in the mid-cycle there is a second phase: a sudden or gradual rise of 0.5 to 1.0 degree to a higher level (usually above 98°), which level is sustained with minor fluctuations for the next twelve or thirteen days, until shortly before the next menstrual period, when it begins to fall. The rise in temperature is due to progesterone, produced after ovulation.

WHAT DOES IT MEAN?

Such a biphasic curve is presumptive evidence that ovulation has occurred. *The exact time at which ovulation occurs cannot be pinpointed by this or by any other known test.* Ovulation is believed to occur in most cases within twenty-four to seventy-two hours of the thermal shift. More specifically, ovulation probably occurs twelve to forty-eight hours between the *last* low point on the graph (not necessarily the lowest) and the first elevation that is sustained.

How many days, then, is a woman fertile each month? Well, let's figure a twenty-eight-day cycle with ovulation approximately midway on day fourteen, and let's allow only three days for sperm survival and only one day for egg survival, though it may be longer for both. Then the fertile period consists of four days. But which four days? That's the unknown.

The reason that ovulation cannot be pinpointed any closer is that the temperature graph at its most reliable is still subject to hormonal fluctuations. For example, if there happens to be an over-production of estrogen in a particular cycle, it will "hold down" the temperature for perhaps two to three days even though ovulation has already occurred. This can be shown by correlating daily temperatures with daily vaginal smears.

For these and other reasons, one can never "predict" from temperature readings when ovulation *will* occur; one can only say in retrospect (if there is a rise) that it has already occurred.

The temperature graph provides the earliest diagnostic sign that pregnancy has actually taken place. That is, if the post-ovulatory basal temperature elevation is continuously maintained for twenty days after the rise, the woman is pregnant. This is one of the happiest uses of the temperature graph in infertility work. The patient is actually the first to know. In fact, even by the eighteenth day of elevation, the diagnosis is almost certain. I have numerous graphs of infertility patients who became pregnant during the course of study, and these "pregnancy graphs" form a particularly special collection. Many show little sketches of smiling faces in place of the dots on the chart, sometimes ending with an explosive "Hooray!" or "We made it!"

HOW TO TAKE THE TEMPERATURE

The doctor will usually explain the procedure, which is quite simple:

1. Shake the thermometer down the night before and put it by the bedside.

2. Put the thermometer under your tongue for five minutes whenever you awake, before you get out of bed or do any other activity. (Read it later if you're sleepy; the reading won't change at room temperature.)

3. Read it to the nearest tenth of a degree (it is helpful but not essential to use a specially graded, easy-to-read basal thermometer which is calibrated only between 97.0° and 100°).

4. If you have a cold or sore throat or are otherwise ill, record that on the chart.

INTERPRETING THE GRAPH

It is up to the doctor to interpret the temperature graph. There are many possibilities. It may be a perfectly normal pattern, with the usual sharp rise and well-maintained elevation until just before menstruation, or there may be a different pattern. For example, there may be only a slight rise, or a poorly sustained one with a tendency to "dip"; or there may be a very slow "staircase" rise, perhaps not as serious as the other patterns mentioned but nevertheless worthy of investigation. Or the rise may be a good one but too short-lasting—perhaps only six to nine days instead of the normal twelve to fourteen days before the onset of the next menstrual period.

The basal temperature graph can therefore show evidence of faulty ovulation, hormonal imbalance, estrogen or progesterone deficiency, or other suspected or unsuspected abnormalities. It also helps to evaluate results of hormonal therapy, given to stimulate ovulation. And it helps the doctor select the day or days for therapeutic husband or donor insemination, when those special procedures are indicated.

It also shows absence of ovulation. When the woman does not ovulate, the temperature curve is no longer biphasic; it is monophasic—that is, there is no shift to a higher level. It is *expectedly* monophasic in adolescent girls before they begin to ovulate, in pre-menopausal women as ovulation begins to falter, and in all men.

The patient should not try to interpret her own graph, for she will find it most frustrating. Every rise can be interpreted as ovulation, only to be disproved the next day. It is a losing battle. The woman should merely take her temperatures according to directions.

WHEN TO STOP

Daily temperature taking is burdensome and should be done for a limited time only. When the woman says that any temperature taking makes her nervous, the husband can often take responsibility by personally placing the thermometer in her mouth when she awakens and then reading it himself. But even this may be too much for a woman who has been to several doctors and has kept graphs for each. Keeping daily temperatures is in itself a singularly unromantic way to start the day, and it isn't that reliable. For the woman who has had enough of temperatures, it is best to stop. Such advice always comes as welcome relief. Besides, no one has ever conceived just by taking temperatures.

9

OVULATION
AND THE "EGG TEST"

In comparison to the mature female rabbit, which ovulates whenever it copulates, the human female is relatively infertile. During her thirty years or so of fertility a woman ovulates once a month—passing a total of about four hundred ova during her lifetime. Moreover, once she conceives, there can be no further ovulation for a long time, at least nine months and more often a year.

OVULATION PROCESS

A human ovum is extruded once a month. However, the ovum does not emerge "naked." It is surrounded by a mass of follicular nutrient cells, the "corona radiata," and this may help the tubal fimbria get a firmer hold on it. Several hours later the ovum loses its corona nutrient cells. It will take another four or five days for the egg to reach the uterus. During this journey it is helped along by the sway of little hairs within the tube and also by the motions of the tubal musculature.

These events, which are nothing short of spectacular, dovetail in such a way as to ensure a favorable environment for the ovum to be fertilized and to help its passive transfer through the tube to its nesting site in the womb at precisely the time when the uterus is prepared for it.

The question is often raised: Does the act of intercourse itself stimulate ovulation? There is no scientific evidence that this is the case in the human. It is the case with certain animals like the female rabbit, which accounts for its unusual fecundity.

MENSTRUATION AND OVULATION

The relationship between menstruation and ovulation has always been a confusing one to the laity. A frequently asked question is, "Can you menstruate without ovulating?" The answer is yes. In such cases, periods are usually, but not always, irregular. Now the other question: "Can you ovulate without menstruating?" The answer is no. If a woman ovulates, she will always menstruate about two weeks later unless pregnancy intervenes.

From the standpoint of fertility one can only say that a woman with normal and regular periods *probably* ovulates regularly, while a woman with grossly irregular cycles is at best ovulating erratically, if at all.

FAULTY OVULATION

A woman may ovulate, yet produce eggs of diminished fertility. We know that *normally* about 15 percent of ova produced by a woman will be completely unfertilizable. It is estimated that perhaps another 25 percent of eggs, when fertilized, will never make it, ending up as very early miscarriages or so-called "silent" abortions in which no period is actually missed. That leaves only about 60 percent of ova for making babies, which explains why even highly fertile women do not necessarily conceive the first month they try; it may take several cycles for one of those better-grade ova to make its appearance.

That's the case with normal egg production. When production of ova is below par, however, an infertility problem often results.

How does a woman know whether or not she is producing eggs of diminished fertility? She doesn't. Her doctor must painstakingly come to that conclusion only after a number of special tests.

SIGNS AND SYMPTOMS OF OVULATION

How does a woman know she is ovulating regularly, or precisely when this event occurs? The only absolutely sure sign that ovulation has definitely occurred is the presence of pregnancy. All other signs and symptoms are presumptive. Let this not imply, however, that such other signs carry little weight: with many of them there is little room for doubt.

Possibly the most interesting subjective symptom of ovulation is so-called mid-month pain, or *mittelschmerz*. This is a characteristic discomfort that many women experience either regularly or sporadically about fourteen days before the expected menstrual period. There may be some premonitory aching for a day or two, then a sudden increase in discomfort in the left or right side of the lower abdomen, usually subsiding in a few hours. It is called ovulation pain, because that is what it is due to. Furthermore, mid-month pain can be correlated with other possible signs of ovulation.

Premenstrual tension is another sympton suggestive of prior ovulation. This annoying syndrome has often been linked with progesterone levels (progesterone can be produced only after ovulation).

However, premenstrual tension has also been related to a number of other complex factors, and its successful management demands individualized therapy.

Some women experience slight staining for a day or two during the mid-cycle. This is also associated with ovulation; at least it is strongly suggestive of it. Incidentally, such mid-month bleeding, when substantial, may account for some of the reported cases of conception occurring during the "menstrual flow," the abundant intermenstrual bleeding being mistaken for such a flow.

Many women also notice an increased slippery, clear nonirritating discharge, something like raw egg white, for several days near the mid-cycle. This slippery discharge originates not in the vagina itself, but from the cervical canal, the neck of the womb. The discharge itself is not specific for ovulation, since it is merely caused by increased estrogen production. However, the appearance of such secretion at that time of month, and its disappearance a few days later, is always strongly suggestive that ovulation has occurred.

Many women can suspect that they ovulate regularly without *any* other signs or symptoms—the mere history of painful periods strongly suggests that ovulation has taken place. Women who do not ovulate generally have painless periods (periods can also be rendered painless by birth-control pills, which inhibit ovulation). However, let it not be inferred that women with painless periods don't ovulate; we know only that women who *do* have pain generally *do* ovulate.

In short, although the tiny female ovum is elusive, its very presence is widely felt by reverberations throughout the body.

TESTS FOR OVULATION

Spinnbarkeit: This is one of the characteristics of cervical mucus, mentioned above. If a doctor puts a drop of such cervical mucus on a glass slide and tries to "stretch" it with tweezers, it will be found to be quite elastic, in that it can be stretched for several inches before snapping back. This elastic property of cervical mucus at the mid-cycle is called *spinnbarkeit*. After ovulation there is a rapid reduction of elasticity to the point that the cervical secretion can be stretched no farther than a drop of water. This change of elasticity, first the build-up and then the decrease, is strongly suggestive of ovulation.

The Fern Test: Still another characteristic of cervical mucus in women who presumably ovulate is the appearance and disappearance of the so-called "fern phenomenon." The test is so named because if a drop of mid-month cervical mucus is spread on a glass slide and allowed to dry, the microscope will show a luxuriant fern-leaf-like pattern. Such ferning begins to appear early in the cycle, reaching a maximum at ovulation time, then gradually disappearing. It is caused indirectly by estrogen stimulation, but actually by the presence of salt in the mucus. For that reason, any salt solution (even a drop of ink) will show the same microscopic picture. While the cyclic fern phenomenon does not clinch the diagnosis of ovulation occurrence, it, too, is strongly suggestive. The presence of staining or cervical infection may interfere with the test.

The so-called glucose *color test* for fertility (ovulation) is typical of the do-it-yourself kits of which there are various types. In my experience, such color tests are generally unreliable.

Another, rather more elaborate method of determining the occurrence of ovulation is by means of daily *vaginal smears*. This is a chore for the woman, who must aspirate some vaginal mucus with a special glass tube each morning, place it on a glass slide, then plunk it into alcohol-ether fixative, and do this for a whole month. However, the results may be helpful in pointing out subtle hormonal changes in the otherwise expected ovulatory pattern.

The *basal temperature graph*, which we have already discussed, is a simpler test. As we have seen, this gives one vital clue, the evidence that ovulation has or has not taken place.

Two of the most reliable tests for the presence and quality of ovulation are the blood progesterone level and the endometrial biopsy ("egg test").

THE ENDOMETRIAL BIOPSY

The endometrial biopsy not only determines that ovulation has (presumably) occurred, but also tests for the quality of the ovum (the ovum itself is unavailable). Eggs of good quality are responsible for good hormonal production, resulting in succulent glands, which provide for an optimum nesting place for a fertilized egg, i.e., for itself. On the other hand, poor-quality eggs are responsible for mediocre hormonal production and the womb lining will show poorly developed glands, with slimmer chances of supporting a fertilized egg.

The test consists of taking a bit of tissue from the lining of the womb a week or more after ovulation is presumed to have occurred and sending it to the laboratory for microscopic examination. Normally, such tissue should show the juicy glands associated with progesterone production; progesterone is produced only after ovulation.

Since the egg test involves scraping tissue from the lining of the uterus, the couple is usually advised to use contraception that particular month; this avoids the remote possibility of interrupting a newly started pregnancy. Interestingly, of several patients who did not report their failure to follow these instructions, some became pregnant during the very cycle in which the biopsy was taken. They carried nicely to term and delivered normal babies. Similar experiences have led some investigators to believe that the procedure may actually *aid* conception by "plowing up the field," as it were, but this is a matter of conjecture. Several intricate studies have shown that the actual chance of interrupting a pregnancy by this procedure is very slim.

ABSENCE OF OVULATION

Faulty egg production is bad enough. More serious is a complete *absence of ovulation*. There are times when lack of ovulation is normal and expected, such as during the years marking the beginning and the end of reproductive life.

What happens when a woman stops ovulating, or never starts? The most noticeable effect is an absence of menstrual periods—but not always, for some women do have periods (usually irregularly) without ovulating.

Sometimes this is revealed unexpectedly. I have in mind one patient, Joan, a twenty-four-year-old secretary who consulted me not for infertility but for contraception. Joan had recently married and, because of religious considerations, wanted to use the rhythm method of birth control. I suggested daily temperatures for a few cycles to find out her "safe period." At her next visit Joan brought in her temperature readings, and there was *no* evidence of ovulation at all. In other words, she was menstruating without ovulating, and was in effect infertile. Naturally she was stunned to hear the news. Obviously rhythm or any other method of contraception would, in this case, have been superfluous.

In her particular case, it turned out that the thyroid gland was primarily at fault. After correction of this deficiency she began to ovulate again and became pregnant shortly afterward, somewhat sooner than originally planned but with considerable relief. She has since had another baby, and has gone on to practice rhythm successfully to date.

In the above case, infertility was discovered incidentally. The patient was having menstrual periods and did not suspect that anything was wrong.

There is no doubt about something being wrong, however, when the woman who has been having menstrual periods suddenly stops. It is an alarming experience, and the most common cause is sudden absence of ovulation.

One of the most common causes of temporary cessation of ovulation and of menstrual periods (amenorrhea) is some emotional shock or tur-

71

moil. It can be almost anything—a death in the family, an unhappy love affair, a mother-in-law coming for a long visit, a mother-in-law coming for a short visit. In such stress situations ovulation may cease for one or more months, but the body usually makes a good recovery when the turmoil is over, and it then resumes normal function.

The mechanism through which the emotions can govern glandular function is discussed in Chapter 12.

Another common cause of sudden absence of ovulation and menstruation is one I frequently see in young women who have just completed a "crash diet," self-imposed and unsupervised. In such cases, periods can be absent for quite a long time, even if the weight is regained. Eventually the body does resume normal function. A marked gain in weight can have the same effect; in addition, the doctor should be on the lookout for emotional problems so often related to obesity.

Any acute or chronic illness can cause cessation of periods; obviously the doctor will direct his attention to the underlying disorder rather than the absence of periods.

HORMONAL FACTORS

The majority of women whose periods stop for reasons other than pregnancy are found to have some sort of hormonal imbalance. The problem for the physician to solve is: Where is the basic defect? Are the ovaries themselves at fault? Or are they being adversely influenced by other glands, such as the thyroid, adrenal or perhaps the pituitary? There are complex hormonal studies and tests to unravel the puzzle and derive a meaningful answer. Specific therapy will depend on that answer.

Sometimes the problem is unexpectedly complex. I recall one patient, Lenore, a thirty-three-year-old woman whose periods had ceased. She was single but nevertheless concerned about her fertility, since she was contemplating marriage within the next year or two. The absence of periods alerted her to the fact that something was wrong, and she came for advice and treatment.

An investigation of her glandular function revealed a high pituitary secretion as seen in menopausal women, when the pituitary tries so hard to stimulate ovaries which are no longer able to respond. In other words, she had *premature menopause,* complete ovarian failure, for which there is no known remedy as far as fertility is concerned. I was therefore unable to restore her reproductive function but did suggest hormonal replacement to avoid some of the symptoms and signs of estrogen deficiency which she had already developed.

THE "FERTILITY PILL" AND PERGONAL

Suppose the diagnostic study reveals that the ovaries themselves are at fault and they are just not producing ova, even though properly stimulated by other glands. Years ago this was a very serious problem. Nowadays there are new therapeutic approaches to help such conditions.

One is the so-called fertility pill (clomiphene citrate). Contrary to popular belief, this substance is not a hormone at all but is a synthetic chemical that is capable of stimulating the ovaries to produce ova in many instances. The mechanism of action is not completely understood. Not all patients with ovulation defects should receive the fertility pill, and the doctor must make an individual judgment as to its possible value.

Although there is a somewhat greater than average chance of twins with the fertility pill (clomiphene), this is not the drug that has been so notoriously publicized in connection with quadruplets and quintuplets. That drug is Pergonal, an injectable hormonal pituitary preparation.

The development of Pergonal has an interesting background. It began with the knowledge that postmenopausal women have a high level of pituitary secretion; this led to the successful isolation of a follicle-stimulating hormone *to help younger infertile women,* a spectacular development in the treatment of certain ovulation problems. This precious pituitary substance is actually extracted from the urine of postmenopausal women. It is therefore known as human menopausal gonadotropin, HMG, or Pergonal. Patients receiving this hormone are mainly those with ovulatory defects due to poor pituitary production, constituting only a small percentage of infertility cases.

This is fortunate, since treatment with Pergonal is very expensive, tedious and unpredictable, even with daily monitoring. Aside from multiple births, there is a substantial risk of overstimulating the ovaries, which can become greatly enlarged. In extreme cases they can rupture and hemorrhage, requiring emergency surgery.

Pergonal alone will not usually induce ovulation, but it has been found that Pergonal and the addition of human chorionic gonadotropin (HCG), easily obtained from the urine of *pregnant* women, constitutes the most potent ovulation stimulant known. Dosage regulation is most important, but even with the best attention the in-.

cidence of multiple pregnancies, as stated, has been high. These include the publicized newspaper stories of quadruplets and quintuplets, always a dramatic occurrence, though not always a happy one, since multiple births mean premature babies with a frequently poor salvage rate.

Research in this field is continuing, and new and better treatments will doubtless be developed as time goes on.

There is one condition that stands apart and is rather special—the so-called hard-shelled ovary. Such ovaries are capable of being stimulated by the woman's own pituitary gland, but the maturing eggs cannot be extruded because of a thick, hard capsule covering the ovaries. A lot of unextruded eggs collect under such a capsule, giving the ovary a characteristic "polycystic" appearance, the so-called Stein-Leventhal syndrome. The best way to be sure of the diagnosis is by direct visualization (described in Chapter 11).

Among the treatments for these hard-shelled polycystic ovaries are cortisone by-products, and the fertility pill (clomiphene). However, if there is no response (i.e., no ovulation) after a few months of such treatment, an operation on the ovaries may produce the desired results. In this procedure "wedges" are removed from both ovaries, and all remaining cysts are obliterated by puncturing. Exactly why this operation should result in the resumption of ovulation in a large percentage of cases is not clear; suffice it to say it does help, and a pregnancy rate of over 50 percent has been reported in several series.

Ovarian polycystic disease is basically a *hormonal* disorder; many patients not only have irregular or absent periods but excessive hair and obesity as well. Women with this disorder who do *not* wish to conceive should be treated with estrogen and progesterone to prevent the progression of the hormonal imbalance.

10

TESTING THE FALLOPIAN TUBES

Since fertilization takes place in the tubes, the first requirement must be an unobstructed passageway from two directions, one for the sperm coming up and the other for the egg coming down. Anything that narrows this passage (which is no wider than a broom straw) can interfere with conception.

The inner lining of the tube is exquisitely delicate, consisting of a velvety surface on which there are countless tiny hairlike structures called cilia. These constantly move in the direction of the uterus, "waving" the egg toward its resting place. It is against this current that the sperm must swim to meet and merge with the egg at the farthest end of the tube.

But what if the ovum can't get into the tube? If the open end of the tube is too narrow, the ovum that is extruded from the ovary that month will simply fall free into the abdominal cavity and wither. The woman will not know that this has happened, for she will feel no different than usual.

The tube itself must also be free to move. Such movement is of two types: one is toward the ovary, the better to receive the ovum; the other, called peristalsis, consists of rhythmic muscular contractions of the tubal wall, which, together with the ciliary action, help move the ovum toward the uterus.

What if the tubes are held down by adhesions—filmy scar tissues? In that case they may not be able to move freely to receive the egg or to propel it properly. Worse still, if any infection or other condition narrows the open ends of the tubes, the ovum cannot even get in, and no pregnancy is possible.

What can one tell about the tubes on physical examination? Normally the tubes cannot easily be felt on pelvic examination. (If they can, that's a clue in itself, usually spelling trouble.) If the history does not disclose any unusual diseases, and the physical examination is negative, how then can one find out whether the tubes are in good shape? There are three diagnostic procedures. They are not overlapping tests, for each gives certain information that the others don't. Together they form a most comprehensive diagnostic triad, and no tube can get a clean bill of health before passing inspection by all three.

THE RUBIN TEST

The most common and familiar of these diagnostic measures is the Rubin test, or tubal insufflation. This consists of passing carbon-dioxide gas slowly and with measured pressure through the tubes by means of a special instrument placed within the opening of the womb. Dr. I. C. Rubin, for whom the test was named, described this procedure sixty years ago, and it is still going strong. A special tracing (kymograph) is usually attached to the apparatus for a permanent record of the pressure readings.

Normally the gas bubbles through the tubes at a certain pressure without undue discomfort. When the patient sits up after the test, she experiences some pain in one or both shoulders as the result of the gas rising under her diaphragm. When she again assumes the reclining position, the discomfort vanishes (since the gas bubble descends), and in another few minutes she can arise comfortably, since by then the gas has been absorbed. Therefore the test need not be uncomfortable.

The initial shoulder pain is essential to prove that one or both tubes are open. The side on which the shoulder pain is felt is determined only by the direction the gas happens to take as it is shunted by the intestines like a pinball machine. One-sided shoulder pain does not mean that only the corresponding tube is open.

Sometimes shoulder pain is not felt immediately but is delayed several minutes or even several hours. When this happens there is a suspicion that gas has passed through the tubes but was trapped in adhesions around them, escaping only much later.

When there is no shoulder pain at all following the test, one must assume that no gas has passed through. Usually the pressure graph will bear this out as well, since it will also show "no passage" despite high pressure. Such a result may be due either to tubal spasm or to actual closure.

Tubal spasm is an interesting phenomenon. Try

feeding spinach to a child who has clenched his teeth in defiance. It is impossible. But you know he doesn't have lockjaw and that the mouth will open under more favorable circumstances, such as when ice cream is offered instead. Much the same can happen to the tubes, but involuntarily. In the first place, the tubes may react unfavorably to having gas "fed" through, and they may understandably clam up during the process. The experienced doctor knows this, and therefore repeats the test under different conditions—for instance, after giving relaxants or injecting an anesthetic into the nerves alongside the uterus. Then, if the initial result was due only to spasm, the repeat test may show an entirely different picture, with gas coming through nicely.

Tubal *closure* is an entirely different matter: the gas test shows no passage, no matter what tricks are tried. Obviously, further investigation is needed.

Somewhere between wide-open and tightly closed tubes, there is an important intermediate area requiring diagnostic acumen. The gas test may indicate that gas has passed through, and shoulder pain follows, but pressure readings don't look right. They are too high or too low, too jerky or not jerky enough. In other words, there is a suspicion that the tubal openings are somehow hampered or constricted. Here, too, further investigation is needed.

THE X-RAY

A second, noncompetitive way of testing tubes is by a special x-ray technique called hysterosalpingography, meaning picture-taking of the inside of the uterus and tubes.

This is obtained by instilling a special dye into the uterus (and, hopefully, through the tubes) and taking x-rays during several stages of the instillation. The uterine part is useful in delineating any abnormalities within the womb itself.

If the uterine opening to the tubes is not blocked, the dye will flow into the tubes and the x-ray will show the entire tubal passageway. Any blockage along this very narrow passage is shown by a stoppage of dye at that point, at the outer end of the tube, in the middle, or wherever it may be. The x-ray, therefore, is helpful in delineating the area of tubal block. If the passageways are clear, the dye will actually spill out, and "free" dye will then be seen outside the tubes in a later x-ray.

Sometimes one or the other of these diagnostic procedures—either the Rubin test, or the special dye and x-rays of uterus and tubes—is in itself therapeutic, as when filmy adhesions are broken up by the pressure of gas or dye and the tubes thereby opened. Sometimes this alone is sufficient to cure the fertility problem.

However, let us assume that there is evidence of partial or complete blockage of the tubes, not remedied by passage of gas or dye through them. What next? If the rest of the infertility studies have shown no other abnormalities to be corrected, attention may be directed to a more detailed investigation of the tubes. The method I shall describe is primarily diagnostic but very often therapeutic as well. It is called endoscopy and is a minor hospital operative procedure requiring an overnight stay. It is discussed in detail in the following chapter.

11

ENDOSCOPY AND
THE SURGICAL TREATMENT
OF TUBAL DISORDERS

Endoscopy is the most revealing of diagnostic procedures for infertility. It is a method by which the doctor can look directly into the pelvis, see all the pelvic organs—the uterus, ovaries and tubes—and test the tubes under direct vision. Consider first the vaginal approach-culdoscopy.

Culdoscopy is done with the patient in the jack-knife (knee-chest) position, which makes the pelvic organs more accessible. Heavy sedation is given and a local anesthetic is injected near the uterus, the combination making the procedure quite painless.

An instrument called the culdoscope is inserted through the back part of the vagina into the pelvic cavity. The instrument (which looks like the cystoscope urologists use to look into the bladder) has a tiny lighted bulb at its end and a system of prisms that enables the doctor to see all angles, like a periscope.

The uterus—its size, shape and position—can be clearly seen; the ovaries are also clearly visible. Finally the tubes are seen, and the doctor notes whether or not they look normal, whether they are free or surrounded by adhesions, whether there are any signs of past infection or of present disorders, such as endometriosis (described on p. 15).

After observation, special blue dye is instilled through the uterus while the tubes are still being observed. The dye can be seen emerging from the tubes (if they are sufficiently open) and the doctor notes whether there is a free spill, a drop-by-drop spill due to constriction, or perhaps no spill at all, with ballooning of the dye just beyond the stricture. *Often a partial constriction can be overcome by exerting extra pressure.*

All this information makes culdoscopy an invaluable procedure in any infertility study. As a matter of fact, even if the gas test and x-ray of the tubes prove "normal," it is possible that the tubes are actually not normal—only culdoscopy can prove it, and has done so on many occasions. Moreover, many cases of so-called "psychological" infertility have simply not withstood the close scrutiny of culdoscopy, which often discloses unsuspected physical causes for infertility. Here is an example.

Sandra and Fred had been to several doctors and they had been told by each that there was "nothing wrong." (Such a problem is always most challenging.) Sandra, who was twenty-five, was about to go to a psychiatrist, and her husband was ready to join her from frustration alone. I looked over the data. There had been quite an extensive study. The sperm were excellent and the postcoital test normal. There was no defect in ovulation and hormone studies were all normal. The

Rubin (gas) test showed good passage under normal pressure with immediate shoulder pain, and the x-rays confirmed the fact that the tubes were apparently normal and open. What was wrong?

Only one procedure had been omitted: culdoscopy. It was possible that culdoscopy would show everything to be normal, in which case this would really be a diagnostic puzzle. No one could say, without taking a look.

Culdoscopy was performed and showed that the tubes, although open, had a peculiar corkscrew shape. Furthermore, although dye did emerge, the tubal ends were narrowed and had a "worm's head" appearance rather than the normal funnel shape. There was no evidence of endometriosis or any other apparent cause to explain the findings. In short, culdoscopy proved there was a physical rather than a psychological basis for this couple's infertility problem.

The therapy chosen for her particular condition was *hydrotubation:* the instillation (in the office) of an antibiotic plus cortisone solution through the tubes. This makes a better "battering ram" than carbon-dioxide gas alone, although gas is also put through as a chaser. This procedure was carried out for three cycles, to further dilate the ends of her tubes. The patient conceived in the third month of treatment. She had a normal pregnancy and delivery.

Laparoscopy is another diagnostic technique for visualizing the pelvic organs. The viewing instrument is placed through a small incision in the abdomen, and gas is pumped in to push other organs aside. Although more elaborate than culdoscopy and requiring general anesthesia, laparoscopy is preferred by many doctors because of their training and because of the usually good visualization obtained, even in the rare case where culdoscopy is not feasible.

Although the procedure used will depend upon the personal preference and experience of the operator, the advantages of *culdoscopy* are that it does not require general anesthesia and that instrumental entry through the vagina is less risky than through the abdomen.

TUBAL SURGERY

When tubal stricture is so severe that it cannot be overcome by office procedures such as hydrotubation, or if pelvic adhesions are so extensive as to make the tubes virtually functionless, more definitive steps are needed. When fertility is otherwise normal, and *if endoscopy has delineated the exact problem,* the tubal surgery may be considered.

Tubal surgery is unlike any other kind in that organs are not removed but rather reconstructed. What is done depends, of course, on the specific problem, but the goal is always to preserve tubal function while eliminating all factors that may hamper it.

The patient should be informed about her chances of success following a tuboplasty, the *only* criterion of success being a live birth. Since such surgery is a last-resort procedure for damaged tubes, the true success rate is not notably high, usually less than 50 percent, largely depending upon the extent of the disorder and other factors.

Surgical techniques include the use of special thin catheters for dilating strictures, extremely thin sutures to hold in place delicate, reconstructed folds, and sometimes plastic prostheses, which must later be removed.

THE WORK-UP

Microsurgery (operating under high magnification) is an exceedingly interesting new technique requiring elaborate apparatus and considerable experience (usually by animal experimentation). It is already considered the procedure of choice in reconstituting tubes that have been ligated, and will undoubtedly have wider application if future statistics show it to be superior to conventional techniques in specific circumstances.

12

EMOTIONAL FACTORS

Emotions can influence reproduction and fertility through intimate association with hormonal function. We have already seen how stress situations can cause the tubes to go into spasm, or cause ovulation to cease altogether.

The mechanism through which the emotions can govern glandular function is via a higher center, the hypothalamus (mid-brain)—the undisputed ruler of the glandular system and the seat of the emotions. When the hypothalamus is disturbed, the whole body is disturbed, and in particular the pituitary, the most important lieutenant of the hypothalamus. Thus, for example, if the pituitary is not working properly, the ovaries get no signals, no eggs mature, no period comes—everything is at a standstill. Then, when the hypothalamus is calm again, and not before, it will signal to the pituitary. Hormonal production will begin again, the ovaries will receive the signal, an egg will mature, the uterus will respond, and the woman will finally get her period.

The situation can be even more complex when

the psychological causes are hidden—as when deep-seated fears of childbirth (or, in men, of causing childbirth) can actually create sexual incapacity, even impotence. Here psychotherapy may be needed to bring the causes into the open— the first step to understanding and, hopefully, to cure.

Take the singular case of a patient I'll call Helen. She had a complete infertility investigation during which no abnormalities were found. At this point, I reviewed her history and background again. She was happily married. She and her husband were eager to have a baby, and she had no reservations about this. But during one consultation she suddenly began to cry and finally admitted she did have a deeply hidden fear. Her sister had died of an incurable blood disorder, but she also happened to be pregnant at the time she died. Helen realized that pregnancy was not the actual cause of death, but she could not remove her gnawing fear that when she herself became pregnant, the same thing would happen to her.

Here, then, was a clue—a conflict between wanting a child and fearing pregnancy. But how did this fear prevent Helen from conceiving? Her records showed two normal tube tests with gas, both done early in the cycle during a time of relatively lessened fertility. I now scheduled a new tube test for the time of maximum fertility— during ovulation. This test revealed the tubes to be "closed"—actually only in spasm, as I knew from her other tests—and repeating the test at a less fertile time of her cycle showed her tubes to be open again.

Together we analyzed the results and discussed her fears, now out in the open. After several consultations with her late sister's internist as well as with her obstetrician, Helen seemed convinced that her sister's death had not, in fact, been caused by pregnancy. She also seemed much more relaxed. However, it took several months longer before her tubes "relaxed" enough to remain open during her fertile time. And still longer, almost six more months, before she finally became pregnant. It was only after her pregnancy was over, and she and her baby were home safe, that she felt her fears completely dissipated.

This is a startling example of infertility caused by emotional factors. It illustrates how the emotions can directly influence physiological functions, in this case causing tubal spasm only when the patient was fertile—that is, vulnerable.

Other ways in which emotional factors can cause infertility have been presented in Chapter 2, in the discussion of "psychological causes."

13

UNSUCCESSFUL
PREGNANCIES

When pregnancy occurs there is usually much
jubilation, but always mixed with a little trepida-
tion—because pregnancy is only the first step,
though a giant one. Happily the majority of
women who conceive will carry nicely to term, but
for some there is disappointment in store.

Several things can happen. There may be a miscarriage (spontaneous abortion), which can occur
early or late. With some women there is a tendency for miscarriages to keep recurring (habitual
abortion). Sometimes the embryo may cease to
grow but not be expelled for many weeks (missed
abortion). Occasionally the fertilized egg can get
stuck in the tube, threatening to rupture (ectopic
pregnancy). And occasionally there are fetal abnormalities, fortunately rare.

"Miscarriage" is the term the layman uses to
describe the birth of a baby too immature to survive. Medical books refer to the occurrence as an

90

"abortion." The mechanism of expulsion of the fetus from the womb is the same as with the full-grown baby, by contractions of the muscular walls of the uterus. But in the case of miscarriage, it is a miniature labor. It does not take as much dilating to expel a small fetus; therefore the labor is much shorter. However, since miscarriage is accompanied by bleeding and much anxiety, the physical discomfort may parallel the mental anguish.

For women who are eager to have a baby, a miscarriage represents a particularly cruel disappointment. One of the first reactions is that of self-blame. The woman torments herself: "What did I do wrong? I was too active. I shouldn't have carried those groceries yesterday. I should not have gone on that trip last week."

Contrary to belief, ordinary (and even extraordinary) activity does not cause miscarriage. This has been shown time and again in various surveys. But a woman who miscarries can always recall some preceding event that she considers responsible. The fact of the matter in cases of miscarriage is that by the time the woman notes bleeding, the embryo has usually been dead for some time, so that events immediately preceding the miscarriage are really inconsequential. If a woman was about to miscarry anyway, any unusual exertion or jolt preceding would naturally be thought of as the cause.

I have found that the most soothing antidote to feelings of guilt about miscarriage is to point out that most cases of spontaneous miscarriage are due to abnormality of the embryo or to faulty implantation. This is a fact, and it is perhaps a small consolation for the woman to know that it is nature's way of getting rid of the imperfectly formed embryo, for there is nothing the pregnant woman fears more than the possibility of a mal-formed baby.

The next question that immediately arises in the case of a woman only threatening to abort is: "If I do not miscarry, will my baby be normal?" The answer is yes, if the pregnancy does go on to full term; the chances of having a normal baby are approximately the same as if no threat had occurred.

A normally implanted pregnancy cannot be shaken loose by running, jumping, or heavy lifting, as many women wishing to abort have discovered. A well-implanted egg with firm moorings in the uterus has been likened to a healthy unripened apple on the tree; a fresh gust of wind will not cause it to fall. However, when anyone who has had a long-standing *infertility* problem finally becomes pregnant, a different set of circumstances prevails. I have found that the degree of anxiety about "holding on" to the baby is such that the woman will usually restrict her own activities, just as she would be extra careful in carrying an extremely fragile object. Such women do not welcome the benefits of unrestricted activity and seem to feel more secure with a few simple restrictions. But even with infertility patients, there is little purpose in maintaining any restrictions beyond three months, since the vast majority of miscarriages occur before the end of the third month.

A word about sexual intercourse. If miscarriage were caused by intercourse, the birth rate would drop to zero. Despite a common and persistent belief that coitus is somehow harmful to pregnancy, there is no scientific evidence to support this. Nevertheless, infertile couples who manage to conceive will often restrict *themselves* from having intercourse "to avoid miscarriage." If such is the frame of mind, I go along with that restriction, but only for the first few weeks, for the simple reason that if the woman does happen to miscarry, she will invariably blame it on the most recent act of coitus. Besides, sex is hardly pleasurable if each act is undertaken with fear and anxiety, and no husband wants to be the "cause" of losing the very pregnancy he so desires. I have tried suggesting partial intercourse for worried infertility couples—that is, coitus without deep thrust, as a compromise, in order not to thwart sex altogether. Often the advice is not taken; anxiety is too great. But gradually, as the end of the third month approaches and all is well, the woman becomes somewhat bolder, and I know that the anxiety is about over when she asks, "Doctor, my husband wants to know if it's all right to . . ."

Miscarriage is relatively common, occurring in about 15 percent of all pregnancies. In addition, definite early miscarriages that would probably have gone unnoticed are often seen during infertility studies when the woman is keeping her temperature record. If she is a few days "late," the graph will indicate whether or not pregnancy has taken place prior to the period.

As mentioned, most miscarriages take place during the first three months, the remainder during the next three. After the sixth month, the birth is called premature if the baby is under five and a half pounds and mature if over.

Where miscarriage is due to defective embryonic formation or faulty implantation, typically the embryo ceases to grow at about six weeks but is retained for another three to four weeks before being expelled. This is why most miscarriages occur around the ninth to eleventh week of pregnancy. Miscarriages occurring significantly later are not likely to be due to a defective embryo but are usually associated with a physical condition in the mother.

What physical condition in the mother can cause a miscarriage? Occasionally fibroids, fibromuscular growths in the wall of the womb, impinge upon the normal growth of the pregnancy and cause it to be expelled. Sometimes a uterus has a misshapen structure which cannot accommodate a growing fetus. On occasion, previous childbirth may have caused deep tears in the neck of the womb, making this area too weak to support a growing fetus and finally causing it to open prematurely in the fifth or sixth month. All of these maternal conditions can be corrected when recognized in the nonpregnant state, so that the *next* pregnancy may proceed normally. However, one of these disorders, the weak cervix, which silently opens, can sometimes be surgically corrected *during* pregnancy if recognized in time.

I shall not easily forget Rhoda, whose case reads like a cliffhanger. At age twenty-six, she had already had three consecutive miscarriages of normal fetuses, all between four and six months. A weak cervix was suspected, the kind that opens up silently. The next time she became pregnant I advised pelvic examination at least once a week to detect any sign of cervical change. Sure enough, at sixteen weeks the cervix began to dilate perceptibly. She was immediately rushed to the hospital and an emergency operation performed, consisting of a deeply placed heavy silk suture encircling the top of the cervix in order to tighten it. She was then examined weekly again. Five weeks after this procedure the cervix unexpectedly began to dilate again, in spite of the suture. She was immediately rushed to the hospital once more. A second operation was done, which encircled and tightened the cervix even higher. At this point she was placed under heavy sedation because of irregular uterine contractions. Gradually the contractions stopped. It was only false labor, a sign of an irritable uterus. The cervix remained closed and she was once more sent home.

The pregnancy continued up to eight months, at which time she suddenly went into spontaneous labor. Once again she was rushed to the hospital, where I quickly removed the suture, since she was in strong labor. Very shortly afterward she was delivered of a four-and-three-quarter-pound normal, healthy boy who, though premature by weight, gained nicely.

Not all such problems end so dramatically or so successfully. A certain amount of luck is needed. If, for example, Rhoda's membranes (bag of waters) had broken during either of her first two hospital admissions, it would have been too late for surgical intervention and she would have inevitably had another miscarriage.

Another case that comes to mind is that of Marion, who had a history of two late miscarriages. Noting that she had fairly large fibroid tumors of the womb, an x-ray was taken, which showed one of them impinging on the lining of the uterus—the type likely to interfere with a growing fetus.

I advised surgical removal of the fibroids before any attempt was made to conceive again. At operation, I did find a large fibroid pressing into the womb, just as the x-ray had indicated. There was also a number of smaller fibroids which I removed as well. Six months later she conceived and, as luck would have it, miscarried again, but quite early this time, the tissue being abnormally developed. In other words, that particular pregnancy was no real test of the new uterine strength.

After what seemed like an endless interval (actually only five months more), she became pregnant again and this time carried beautifully right into the ninth month, at which time I did an elective Caesarean section because of the known surgical scar from the previous operation. The baby, a girl, weighed seven and a half pounds. Marion, who has since moved, sends me a greeting card every year enclosing a photo of the "baby," now long grown up.

It is a myth that miscarriages are more common at the time of the expected menstrual period. There is simply no scientific evidence to support this popular belief. It is also a myth that pelvic examination will cause miscarriage or accelerate it. The importance of a pelvic examination when a woman thinks she may be aborting is to determine whether the miscarriage is inevitable or not, since therapy will depend upon the specific diagnosis.

A miscarriage is considered definite if the woman has passed any fetal or placental tissue. If there is uncertainty about such passage during early pregnancy, a miscarriage is still considered inevitable if the cervix is found to be open. In such cases there will no doubt be bleeding and cramps, and it is best to clean out the uterus by curettage or suction, a minor hospital procedure in which the fragments are removed from the uterine lining.

If, however, the woman has not passed any tissue and the cervix remains closed, the miscarriage is only threatening. The management of such a delicate condition depends upon the doctor and the patient, there being no standardized proper treatment. Many doctors impose no restrictions at all, letting nature take its course, and they report results as good as others who prescribe all sorts of hormones, sedatives and rest. Obviously it is not a settled subject.

In my own practice I handle each problem individually, since each woman's needs, fears and anxieties vary. Since the use of hormones during pregnancy is so controversial, because of possible deleterious effects on the fetus, the question hardly arises any longer. (Most patients would reject it even if offered.) Strict bed rest is not advised, but some limitation of strenuous physical activity is, if only to minimize the inevitable feelings of guilt that would arise should miscarriage follow. Admittedly it is difficult to foretell which threatening cases are doomed, no matter what the treatment. But for those hanging in the balance, so to speak, I prefer to give at least some emotional support whenever possible.

A knotty problem is presented by the patient who miscarries several times in a row. If she has had three or more successive miscarriages, she is known in medical circles as a "habitual aborter." Such patients deserve the most meticulous investigation *prior* to conceiving again, since they are understandably reluctant even to try. This investigation should include a search for hormonal deficiencies, anatomic defects, constitutional and nutritional factors, subnormal sperm and psychogenic factors.

The hormones in question are estrogen, progesterone, and thyroid. Anatomic defects are demonstrated by special x-rays. In addition, if the woman has a retroverted (tipped) uterus, it is moved forward and held in place with a pessary. If it cannot be budged at all, an operation is done to bring it forward, one of the few valid reasons for uterine suspension. If tests show the cervix to be anatomically weak and the patient has had typical late miscarriages, an encircling operation may be performed to tighten this weakness.

The role of subnormal sperm in the causation of habitual abortion is controversial. While no conclusions can be drawn, every effort should be made to bring the quality of sperm to an optimum level.

The Rh blood factor plays no role in *early* miscarriage, whether single or repeated. In the most severe form of Rh problems there is difficulty toward the end of pregnancy, with intrauterine death or premature labor; the fetus will be found to have Rh disease, making the diagnosis apparent. New procedures, such as analyzing the amniotic fluid and giving the fetus transfusions while in utero, have made it possible to save some of the babies who would ordinarily not survive.

A known method of preventing Rh disease will unfortunately not help women who are *already* Rh-sensitized, but will probably make the disorder obsolete in the future. The unsensitized Rh-negative mother who has delivered an Rh-positive infant is simply given an injection of Rh immunoglobulin shortly after giving birth. This prevents her from later producing antibodies that could attack future Rh-positive infants. (It is also given after miscarriage.)

Constitutional and nutritional factors, if poor, should be improved. A well-balanced diet, adequate vitamin intake, avoidance of excess exposure to drugs, alcohol or tobacco, and release from stress by adequate rest and relaxation are all important in the treatment of habitual abortion. Finally the many reports of the successful treatment of repeated miscarriage by nothing more than tender loving care speak strongly for an emotional component which must always be kept in mind.

UNSUCCESSFUL PREGNANCIES

Sometimes the embryo dies, the uterus fails to grow, but miscarriage does not immediately take place; in fact, many weeks can go by. The woman herself is usually unaware of it; it is discovered by the doctor in his routine examination. This is known as a missed abortion. Although such pregnancies are exceedingly vexing to the patient, many doctors advise leaving them alone, as sooner or later spontaneous miscarriage is likely to occur with a great deal less difficulty than if induced. Other doctors prefer to take a more active role in terminating pregnancy.

Undoubtedly the most dramatic complication of pregnancy is an ectopic (misplaced) pregnancy. This occurs when a fertilized egg is lodged in an abnormal location, usually the tube. Although early symptoms may include pain in the side and bleeding, the symptoms are often atypical enough to make it a treacherous condition. Moreover, since the pregnancy cannot expand in such a constricted environment, it may rupture the tube, resulting in internal bleeding that requires emergency surgery. Even without rupture, once the diagnosis is definitely made, surgery is performed to remove the abnormally lodged pregnancy before rupture. Often the affected tube is removed in its entirety; the patient can become pregnant through the other tube in the future. Sometimes, if the ectopic pregnancy is not too large (and, because of infertility, one desires to be as conservative as possible), the pregnancy alone may be removed from the tube, leaving the tube intact after reconstructing it. Results are quite unpredictable. I remember Vera, a colonel's wife, who consulted me many years ago at an Army base. I diagnosed an ectopic pregnancy and removed the affected tube. She was subsequently able to have three normal children with her one remaining tube—no infertility problem there.

In contrast, I can cite one of my most discouraging cases. When Katherine first consulted me she had already had one tube removed some years earlier because of an ectopic pregnancy, then had difficulty becoming pregnant again. After some tests and treatment she finally conceived, only to develop an ectopic pregnancy in her one remaining tube! Since this tube represented her only chance at future fertility, I chose to remove just the misplaced pregnancy, then reconstructed the tube, leaving it in place. It took almost two years before she conceived again. Unfortunately she developed another ectopic pregnancy in the previously operated-on tube, which actually ruptured before she could get to the hospital (there is a statistically high likelihood of such an occurrence). This time I removed the tube, which was a "blowout" and unsalvageable, and so after three ectopic pregnancies she is destined to remain infertile.

On a happier note, I can cite a rather unusual case. Laura, aged twenty-five, had been married five years and had a three-and-a-half-year-old daughter. She was very eager to have another child. At the time she consulted me she gave a history suggestive of a left ectopic pregnancy. Pelvic examination was made more difficult because of extreme tenderness and discomfort. During one examination I thought that she might have a twisted left ovarian cyst rather than an ectopic pregnancy. A few hours later, at reexamination, it felt more like a uterine fibroid, perhaps with degeneration, which can also cause a great deal of pain. In any event, her pain became so severe that exploratory surgery was inevitable. At operation, she was found to have all three conditions! She had a good-sized ovarian cyst on the left side, which had twisted and become hemorrhagic. She also had a good-sized fibroid on the posterior surface of the uterus. Finally, she had the suspected original diagnosis, a small but treacherous ectopic pregnancy lodged in the left tube, with impending rupture. With the removal of these pathological conditions, she made an uneventful recovery and a few months later conceived through the other tube, and carried the baby very nicely.

The possibility of a silent, treacherous, *unruptured* ectopic pregnancy has always been a source of great concern and anxiety to both patient and doctor. Recent advances in medical technology, however, have done much to diffuse this worry.

An extremely sensitive blood test for pregnancy, known as a radioreceptor assay (RRA), *if negative,* almost certainly rules out the possibility of *any* pregnancy, including an ectopic. If positive, a sonogram (sound-wave picture) can often delineate whether or not there is evidence of a pregnancy within the uterus or, if not, whether there are any suspicious shadows in the tubal area. Finally, if an unruptured ectopic pregnancy is suspected on laboratory or clinical evidence, a "peek-in" by laparoscopy is warranted and, if confirmed, the patient is already in position for prompt surgical removal.

14

ONE-CHILD STERILITY

One of the most perplexing and exasperating types of infertility is that which occurs after a first child has been conceived with no difficulty. There is always a special note of frustration in the questions that the doctor knows he will be asked: "What can be wrong? We're the same two people and nothing has changed since three years ago, when I became pregnant practically the first month we tried."

The story is a familiar one. Some women conceive once and then have difficulty in becoming pregnant again. Nothing has changed on the surface, but obviously something *has* changed and is interfering with conception, or else pregnancy would have taken place just as easily as before. The problem is called "secondary infertility" or "one-child sterility."

The feature that is different is precisely the fact that the woman *has* given birth before, for even the most normal pregnancy and delivery can give rise to future difficulty.

One of the most common ways in which childbirth can affect future fertility is by causing a low-grade, imperceptible inflammation of the tubes, which results in their becoming slightly "glued" at their ends. Every delivery opens the normally germ-free uterine and tubal environment to bacteria from the outside. If microscopic sections are taken of the tube a few days after normal delivery, one can almost always demonstrate some evidence of a slight inflammatory process. Most of the time the tubes are able to handle this very well, and soon the tissues are as good as new. However, in a significant number of cases, there is some reaction at their outer, funnel-shaped opening. The fringes in this area become glued together just enough to interfere with an egg getting into the tube, and that's often the whole extent of the problem.

To make the diagnosis, a simple gas-insufflation test is done in the office. The increased pressure required before passage is a clue that there probably is (or was) partial narrowing at the tubal ends. Subsequent easy passage of gas indicates that the obstruction has been overcome. If there are no other impediments, conception usually follows soon afterward.

Another way in which previous childbirth can interfere with future fertility is by its effect on the cervix, the neck of the womb. Often there is a chronic infection set up in this region as a result of a normal delivery, simply because of a greater susceptibility of the cervix to local bacteria after childbirth. This sort of infection is not at all detrimental to general health; its importance is mainly in reference to fertility. The diagnosis is made by visual inspection of the cervix and examination of its secretions. More specifically, the after-intercourse test shows that the sperm are having difficulty traversing the thick, inhospitable mucus. Treatment consists of clearing up the cervical infection.

If this proves to be chronic and prolonged, and there is much eagerness to conceive as quickly as possible, the cervix may be bypassed by inseminating the husband's semen by a special technique.

A patient whom I'll call Barbara had a little girl three years old and had been trying almost two years unsuccessfully to conceive again. Her physical examination proved perfectly normal. She did not complain of any unusual discharge. I checked out her husband's semen, which was excellent. Examination of the cervix revealed no obvious infection and the post-coital test showed good sperm penetration. I decided that it must be a tubal problem, but I was wrong. Gas passed through easily without undue pressure.

It took a while to get the answer, which was revealed by other tests. It turned out that the quality of Barbara's ova was not as good as previously, probably from a hormonal imbalance which may follow any upheaval such as pregnancy. She was given medication to improve the quality of ovulation, plus supportive hormonal therapy after ovulation and she conceived in the third cycle of treatment.

Doris' case was different. She had a four-year-old boy and had been unsuccessfully trying to conceive again for two years. She had been to several doctors who had found "nothing wrong." Their tests had shown that her tubes were open and her husband's sperm were normal; the after-intercourse test had shown many motile sperm at the opening of the womb. It was this last detail that provided the clue I was looking for—I wondered whether sperm would be found not only at the opening but *throughout* the length of the cervical canal as far as, and including, the uterine cavity. Often there is an area of inflammation or congestion deep within the cervix which prevents passage of those very sperm hovering in such large numbers at the opening of the womb.

This was precisely the problem with Doris. In another after-intercourse test, I found that the mucus high in the cervix was effectively filtering out the sperm—and of the many present at the opening, only a few got any higher, and they looked rather sluggish.

It took several months to clear up this inflammation and thus improve the secretions. A later test revealed many active sperm at all levels of the cervix and also within the uterus. Unknown to both Doris and myself at the time of this test, she was well on her way to becoming pregnant, for she missed her very next period. I delivered her of another boy some nine months later, and she has since had still another child—a much-desired girl—without further difficulty.

Some couples with one-child sterility feel a bit greedy about complaining too loudly of their plight. "We should be thankful for the one we have" is the way they usually express it.

Actually, the frustration can be just as intense as when wanting a first child. At the same time, such couples have reason to feel more optimistic, since the mere fact that they already have a child demonstrates that they had good fertility at one time, and hopefully it can be retrieved.

15

THE IMPACT OF INFERTILITY ON MARITAL AND SEX LIFE

A couple that has been trying unsuccessfully to have a baby experiences many moods. One is frustration: "Why does it have to be me?" Another is anger: "Why can't our friends, neighbors and relatives leave us alone? How can they be so tactless as to keep asking us when we're going to have a baby?" Another is fear: "I'd hate to go through all those tests—I hear some of them are absolute agony." There is also resentment and envy and guilt: "What did we do wrong? Who's to blame?"

Blame! It is most important for the husband and wife not to look upon each other as being at fault in any way. The barren marriage is discouraging enough without adding such needlessly destructive attitudes. There is no fault, no blame. Infertility is always a dual problem, since it concerns two people. Chances are that several causes will be uncovered, and it is known that the husband contributes in some measure to almost half the cases. But even if it turns out that one partner has the predominant deficiency, the problem is still bilateral in that it is the couple's *combined* fertility that counts.

The first thing an infertile couple should face is the fact that they are in this together and that they need each other's support in every way. The wife needs desperately to know that her husband does not consider her any less feminine because of her inability to conceive. The husband needs equal reassurance that he is no less masculine for whatever role he plays in their joint problem.

Yet I have seen time and again how infertility can mar a previously good marital and sex life. The worst part is that most of the punishment is self-inflicted and due to misinformation or poor advice.

"—and we've been trying so hard, Doctor!"

When a couple tells me that (and I hear it often), it bothers me because I know what is happening to that couple and to their marriage.

It's usually the wife who offers the information. The husband will nod. Both look miserable.

Any couple worried about fertility already has a strain in their marriage. Whenever a basic human need, such as parenthood, is frustrated, it is understandably a blow to one's self-image. There is often apt to be resentment on the part of the husband or wife for absence of children. If the husband is told his sperm are "weak," it is a threat to his masculinity. It is equally threatening for a wife to learn that her own fertility is less than normal. Both become jittery, overanxious, depressed.

But now a curious thing happens. They begin to wonder about timing. The theme is always the same, though the variations are different. With one couple, it is intercourse every night during

THE WORK-UP

the fertile period. With another, it is every night throughout the month—or whenever her temperature drops, which can also turn out to be daily or every other day.

I could list a dozen more such rules just by going through my case files, but they all have a similar pattern, which is sex on schedule.

Sometimes the instructions are imposed by well-meaning doctors. Often the pattern is established by the wife herself who thinks it can "improve our chances." I have yet to see it imposed by the husband.

He wants to have a baby as much as she does, but he has his limits. "What is it this time?" he asks. "Your temperature? The calendar? A full moon?" Accused of sarcasm and not "cooperating," the husband is ready to give up—emotionally, that is. He wants to help but he can't keep up under pressure. The sad result may be the development of impotence.

His wife is in no frame of mind to understand. They quarrel. The marriage begins to falter.

Fictional? Not at all. It happens to the nicest people.

The really surprising thing about all this is that so many couples are willing to believe or are led to believe that years of infertile marriage can be explained simply by "poor timing." Possibly a protective psychological mechanism operates, making it easier to accept a simple (if illogical) explanation rather than to face a more complex or serious one.

Even so, I have found that it always comes as a relief to the wife when I tell her that temperatures need not be taken month after month. I consider them a diagnostic tool for the physician—and in any case, we have seen that temperature shifts do not necessarily coincide with ovulation, and therefore should not be used arbitrarily as a guide for coital timing. Above all, I emphasize that *incorrect timing is not a common cause of long-standing infertility.*

The husband, in turn, is invariably grateful to learn that by far the best "guide" for coital frequency is mutual desire, and that sex on schedule serves no useful purpose whatsoever. He is likely to have thought so all along but did not wish to seem uncooperative by not following "doctor's orders" or his wife's intuition.

There is another kind of coital regulation which is often imposed. It is commonly believed that prolonged periods of abstinence help to "save up" the sperm when they are subnormal. This may induce severe conflict in the husband. He does not wish to seem uncooperative; yet the knowledge that his sperm are "weak" depresses him and interferes with his sexual performance. If upon this is imposed the additional burden of abstinence, it deprives the couple of normal sex and adds a source of frustration which often leads to marital tension. I hope that all such couples will have learned from this book that abstinence is *not* likely to improve sperm quality or chances of conception.

There are also instances in which the wife becomes unresponsive and frigid, due to marital tensions resulting from infertility. (If there is no sex, she can hardly be blamed for not conceiving, is her underlying subconscious thought.) This attitude, of course, is also one which must be brought out and corrected by the perceptive physician.

Special methods of treatment may add considerably to the general strain. For example, therapeutic insemination of the husband's sperm requires repeated masturbation or withdrawal, an un-

welcome chore at best. Donor insemination requires less of the husband physically, but more
emotionally.

Should pregnancy take place after prolonged
infertility there is the further tendency on the
part of the couple to worry lest sexual relations
"disturb" the embryo, a fear unfortunately too often reinforced by the doctor.

One can readily see how an infertility problem
can profoundly disturb a marital relationship, and
how vital the role of the doctor is in preventing or
alleviating such disturbance. In the average infertility case, it is well for the anxious, self-blaming
wife to keep in mind that emotional tension may
well be the result of infertility, not the cause of it.
This attitude alone helps decrease tension. One
might also point out that countless "nervous"
women reproduce at will.

It is important for the physician treating the
infertile couple to appreciate fully the delicate
sensibilities involved. Such couples place their full
trust in the doctor, who should help dissolve inhib-
itory forces.

When I see a particularly frustrated and anxious couple, I usually ask them: "What is your
greatest anxiety, your worst fear?"

They will usually say that it would be failure in
their efforts to have a baby.

I then ask: "Have you faced this possibility
squarely?" They usually have not. I urge them
strongly to do so—for once they have faced the
worst possibility, anxiety is lessened and there is
more room for optimism.

It is understood that the husband and wife embarking on an infertility work-up are not doing it
for pleasure. It is not their first choice as to how
to have a baby. They are undergoing the work-up
together, and they should not permit it to inter-

fere with their normal day-to-day relationship. Above all, they are embarking on it with the full realization that, if they are successful, the rewards are well worth the effort.

Part Three

AFTER THE TESTS: REAPPRAISAL

16

WHEN TO REEVALUATE
YOUR INFERTILITY PROBLEM

An average infertility study may take only three
to four months. In many instances the couple explain that they have already been to several doctors and have had numerous tests. In that case,
the consultant reviews what has already been
done and decides whether any tests should be repeated—explaining why—and whether new tests
are indicated. In any event, at the end of any infertility study, it is advisable for the physician to
have a conference with the couple to explain the
results, his plan of therapy, and the chances of
success.

How long should the couple wait, then, before
seeking a second (or third or fourth) opinion?
Obviously this will depend upon the nature of the
problem, the particular prognosis given, and, of
course, their confidence in the physician. In general, six to twelve months is a reasonable time to
allow for diagnosis and correction of abnormalities, and to expect a favorable outcome, if it is to

occur—or at least to receive a reasonable explanation if it does not. Often doctors themselves will be the first to advise the couple to seek another opinion and will suggest the names of other consultants.

The main question is: *Has the couple had the benefit of all possible diagnostic procedures and treatments?* The answer must be No if culdoscopy or laparoscopy (direct visualization of the pelvic organs) has not been done.

The thoroughness of an infertility study depends upon the care with which new knowledge is included and applied.

ALLERGY AND INFERTILITY

One such area of relatively new knowledge has to do with immunology (allergic reactions) as it relates to infertility. This is still controversial and not well understood. According to the work of some investigators, the wife can become "allergic" to her husband's sperm. This should not be confused with the difficulties that sperm may encounter from unfavorable secretions in the cervix due to inflammatory or hormonal conditions. In fact, the after-intercourse test may show a normal result in some cases of sperm allergy.

The mechanism of sperm allergy is poorly understood, as is the entire field of immunology. One popular theory is that the wife has gradually developed circulating antibodies against her husband's sperm which may render the sperm ineffectual. There is a special test that notes whether the wife's blood serum causes clumping of the husband's sperm, indicating a high antibody level.

Some studies have shown that such high antibody levels can be reduced by preventing exposure in these women to their husband's semen by abstinence or the use of condoms for about six months. Subsequently such women may become pregnant upon resuming unprotected coitus.

There are several other theories regarding the mechanism of allergic reduction of fertility, including interference with implantation of the fertilized ovum, incompatibility of blood types, and others even more complex.

The allergy concept is actually not a new one and has an interesting history. About a hundred years ago Darwin suggested that infertility may be related to sexual promiscuity in women due to exposure to the semen of many different men. Very little was published on the subject after that, but in 1958, Gebhard and co-workers made the observation that prostitutes are surprisingly infertile. This led more recently to the question as to whether the reputed infertility in prostitutes might be at least partially explained on an immunological (allergic) basis. A study was undertaken by Schwimmer and co-workers, who found that among forty-eight imprisoned prostitutes there was a 70 percent incidence of antisperm antibodies, as compared with 20 percent in a controlled group of unmarried single women. This in no way implies that women with sperm antibodies are promiscuous. The agglutination reaction is a very nonspecific one. In fact, a positive allergy response can be found in virgins, indicating that there are other substances besides sperm antibodies which will give a positive test.

There is much continuing research in this complex field, and obviously much more is needed.

OTHER POSSIBLE CAUSES OF INFERTILITY

Endometriosis has been mentioned elsewhere (p. 15) and should be considered in all patients with a "normal" infertility investigation. The condition can be confirmed only by direct vision. Treatment includes the use of steroids, such as contraceptive pills, or synthetic male hormones, to suppress ovulation and menstruation ("false pregnancy"). In more severe cases, or in instances where its effect upon the tubes is too constricting, surgery is required.

Mycoplasms are tiny, bacterialike organisms believed by some to play an obscure role in some cases of infertility and habitual abortion. However, the role of "T-mycoplasma" in infertility is still an enigma. No well-controlled studies have conclusively demonstrated such a role. Nevertheless, if such organisms are cultured either in the wife's cervical secretions or the husband's semen, therapy is relatively innocuous and may be worth while in patients with persistent or unexplained infertility. Both husband and wife should be simultaneously treated with high doses of tetracycline or a similar compound and then recultured.

Uterine anomalies include congenital abnormalities in shape, such as a womb with two cavities. Such a uterus may be associated with multiple miscarriages, and can usually be corrected by a surgical "unification" procedure.

Intrauterine adhesions may be related to too-vigorous curettage or severe infection. As with uterine anomalies, the diagnosis can be made on x-ray or by looking directly into the uterus with a hysteroscope.

Hysteroscopy is thus another form of endoscopy, which has received relatively recent attention. The indications for this procedure for *infertility* (such as detection of intrauterine disorders or defects) are limited in that these diagnoses can easily be made with other, more familiar procedures.

17

WHEN IT'S TIME TO FACE THE FACTS

One of the things that all women understandably worry about when confronted with infertility is their age. "Time is running out" is the way many women put it, when referring either to their actual age or to the fact that the chances of pregnancy seem unattainable. Sometimes it *is* too late, and the patient must so be told.

In other situations, age may play no role in a generally pessimistic outlook. If the doctor has come to the conclusion that the prognosis is extremely poor, he must be candid in explaining the facts to the couple. There are some conditions—not many—that cannot be remedied.

It is then the physician's duty to help the couple make an emotional adjustment. Advice and help in adopting a child has been the best therapy for many such couples. For others, when the sterility is solely the husband's, donor insemination is a possibility.

The choices are completely dissimilar. To take

just one aspect, an adopted child should eventually be told of his status. In contrast, a baby conceived as the result of donor insemination is, in all eyes, a child of the marriage, and need never be told otherwise.

A discussion of both of these possibilities follows in the next chapter.

18

ALTERNATIVES FOR
THE INFERTILE

THERAPEUTIC DONOR
INSEMINATION

The public at large is understandably hazy about donor insemination. Ask the man in the street about it and he may shrug his shoulders and mention something about "test-tube babies." Not much lay literature exists about the subject; yet it is estimated that thousands of babies have been born as a result of this procedure, and the number is rapidly growing each year.

The reason few people are acquainted with the details of this type of therapeutic insemination is that relatively few have had to come to grips with it. It requires a rather special set of circumstances. One indication, as mentioned, is that the husband must be sterile or so infertile as to be clinically sterile. But there are other indications for donor insemination. For example, if the husband's genetic history is so abnormal that he is unwilling to perpetuate his genes, donor insemination may be considered after consultation with a geneticist. It may also be considered if the couple has already had abnormal offspring stemming from recessive genes likely to produce future congenital defects.

The background of donor insemination is most interesting. The procedure is well known in veterinary medicine, where animal husbandry has developed it into a constructive science for the breeding and improvement of the stock. In humans the pioneer work was done (in secrecy at the time) by Dr. Robert L. Dickinson as far back as 1890. He was one of the first to recognize the therapeutic value of the method; he pressed for its practice and lived to see its acceptance as a recognized therapeutic procedure. It was my privilege to have known this remarkable man, who has also led the way in many other fields of social and sexual health.

Donor insemination is, therefore, no new "fad" but a definite medical procedure which physicians have been performing for many decades in this and many other countries. Nevertheless the procedure is still shrouded in uncertainties, largely because there was no law in any of our states either specifically permitting or prohibiting it until 1967, when a law was enacted in Oklahoma. This is the first statute in any state specifically conferring legality on the use of donor insemination to achieve pregnancy, and spelling out the rights of children conceived in this way. Physicians would certainly welcome laws in other states.

The only other local ordinance implying judicial acceptance of donor insemination exists in New York City. Here, the health department has a specific regulation about donor insemination in Section 112 of the sanitary code adopted in 1947, pertaining to checking the health and other qualifications of a semen donor.

The Oklahoma law would do well to serve as a model for other states. However, the absence of such laws has thrown the burden of resolving legal difficulties on the courts. In general, the majority of such decisions have been favorable to donor insemination. Perhaps the most important was the Sorensen decision in 1967, rendered by the California Supreme Court. After a divorce, the father, Sorensen, refused to support a child which his wife had conceived by donor insemination (to which the husband had consented in writing). Reversing a decision of the Court of Appeals, the California Supreme Court held the defendant to be the legal father and stated that "A reasonable man who, because of his inability to procreate, actively participates and consents to his wife's artificial insemination . . . knows that such behavior carries with it the legal responsibilities of fatherhood." The court also noted the absurdity of considering insemination an "adulterous" act and supported the legitimacy of any offspring so conceived. However, the opinions expressed were *in dicta* and therefore not intended to be binding in other cases. Most cases reaching the courts arrive at similar decisions: in one particular case, the court ruled that the husband had visitation rights, just as though he were the natural parent; in another instance it stated that "When a child is born within a marriage by whatever method, there is a legal presumption that both marriage partners are his parents."

Even to consider donor insemination as "adultery" is to formulate an entirely new meaning for the word. For example, the concept becomes absurd if the insemination is performed by a female physician.

Aside from legal opinions, the religious viewpoint is of interest. In general, it can be said that most Protestant and Jewish denominations in this country approve or at least condone this procedure, while the Catholic Church rejects it. The Orthodox Jewish view is of interest because while it opposes the practice, it recognizes children born of the procedure to be legitimate; nor is the wife considered to have committed adultery, since there was no guilty intent. The views of most Protestant churches have not been officially expressed. The United Presbyterian Church, however, in its 1962 report on responsible parenthood, discusses the question as follows: "To discover [in donor insemination] an act of adultery— though there is no coitus—is certainly to give the word a meaning that it does not have in the New Testament."

I can think of no medical procedure more emotionally delicate than donor insemination. It places an unusual responsibility on the physician, a responsibility not only to the couple involved but also to a child yet unborn. In my experience, couples who have become parents as a result of donor insemination are among the happiest and the most grateful, often returning a second time. But this is largely because of the careful screening that must be done before the procedure can be seriously considered.

In the first place, the desire for donor insemination should stem from the couple. Moreover, husband and wife must each individually prefer this method to adoption. I make it a point to obtain their separate views and to see if either has any reservations. If there is any hesitancy, I recommend waiting.

Sometimes I discover that the husband does not actually prefer this procedure but wants it for the sake of his wife because "she is so eager to have a baby." This is not a solid enough reason to proceed, as it may lead to resentment at some later time. The same holds for a wife who is personally lukewarm to the idea but wants it "because it will bolster my husband's ego." She must want it herself and he must want it himself, not just for the sake of the other.

Furthermore, the marriage must have good stability before the procedure can be considered by the conscientious physician. The doctor should not knowingly attempt to "save" a shaky marriage in this way, for it is far too great a burden to place on any child. Similarly, if the couple requesting donor insemination has been married only a few months, it is best to wait longer, until it is evident that the marriage is indeed on firm ground.

It is likewise inadvisable to accept a couple for this procedure too soon after the diagnosis of the husband's sterility. Such a verdict comes as a shock to any man, and he must be given time to recover emotionally. If the husband has any sperm at all, he is also told that although it is unlikely, there is always the *possibility* that his wife may become pregnant from his own sperm. It can be emphasized that all sperm pictures show considerable variability and while a very poor semen is not expected to change to very good, there is just that outside chance that a slight improvement will coincide with an unusually fertile egg.

It is apparent that the physician's interview with the couple interested in donor insemination must be in great depth in order to weed out all except those genuinely eager for this help. Only after thoroughly exploring the attitudes and reactions of each partner can a meaningful decision be made.

After a couple has been accepted as suitable for this therapy, further details are discussed. I first ask whether anyone (other than doctors who have been treating the couple) is aware of their plan. It is essential that no one else should have knowledge of it for the sake of the baby yet unborn. In most cases they have not discussed their plan with anyone else.

If the husband or wife has confided in a friend or relative that donor insemination is contemplated, I then suggest that the confidence be "reversed." That is, I advise that the person or persons be casually told that the donor plan is being abandoned in favor of some "new treatment" for the husband which will, hopefully, enable him to produce sperm or improve those he has. This is to insure that the husband be established as the father in all eyes, in case the wife does conceive. To repeat, any child resulting from donor insemination is a child of the marriage and never need be told otherwise.

The question of the "legality" of donor insemination often comes up during the interview. My answer is quite simple: There is no legal problem unless one is created by the husband or wife.

In the office, the only paper involved is a "consent" form explaining the procedure, which is signed by the couple.

Naturally the couple want to know about donors, how they are selected and so on. I explain that donors are chosen from among medical students, interns, or residents of the various hospitals in the city. Aside from being of good fertility, each donor's genetic background and physical characteristics are known. This last is particularly important, since an attempt is made to match the physical characteristics of the donor to those of the husband. For example, if the husband is tall with light hair and blue eyes, a donor of similar appearance is chosen, particularly if the wife also has blue eyes.

If the donor matches the husband's blood type, that is preferred. However, a donor who physically resembles the husband but whose blood type is different is preferable to one who has the same blood type but does not share the same resemblance. At the same time, the wife's Rh factor must also be considered. In the event that she is Rh negative, only Rh negative donors are used, in order to avoid any future incompatibilities.

The donor must remain forever anonymous, his identity in any given instance being known only to the physician doing the insemination. Such anonymity is assured by having the semen specimen delivered to the office within an hour by messenger; the donor himself never appears.

If the husband has any sperm at all, the couple will often ask whether it will be mixed with the donor's semen on the theoretical possibility that it will be one of the husband's sperm that will cause the conception. Some twenty years ago I used to do this, but then decided on a different method, which spares the husband the time, effort and tiresome chore of producing a specimen every time his wife is inseminated. An easier method of "mixing" his sperm with the donor's is simply to advise the couple to have intercourse the same night after donor insemination is done. Without exception, husbands have been grateful for this advice, which is far less burdensome and so much more natural.

In written correspondence or in telephone conversations the word "insemination" is never used—just the term "treatment." An appointment is given for a "treatment" on a certain day at a certain hour, and the wife knows what it means.

The procedure actually consists of instilling the donor's semen just within the entrance of the womb at the most fertile time of cycle. The wife keeps a temperature graph and is treated one or more times depending upon the fluctuations in the graph, an arrow on the chart marking the day or days of treatment. (This is a nonspecific sign and could represent other kinds of therapy.)

As might be expected, if the wife is of normal fertility, results are excellent, since the male factor is of unusually high quality. Of those women who conceive with donor insemination, about two thirds become pregnant within the first three cycles. It is for this reason that the wife is not put through any "tests" prior to insemination, since her fertility has never really been tested in her marriage. Only if there is something in the history or physical examination to warrant it, or if pregnancy fails to take place within two or three months, is there an attempt to assess the wife's fertility and begin to look for impeding factors.

Unquestionably the strongest advocates of donor insemination (if they were free to speak) would be those couples who have had babies resulting from this procedure. Many years of follow-up, and the many couples who repeat, attest to the fact that this method of treatment fulfills a vital need.

Unfortunately, only large-sized communities have the resources necessary for anonymity and the selection from a wide variety of donors. Therefore those who live in smaller communities are unable to receive help unless they can afford to travel considerable distances to the larger cities for donor insemination. Doctors who specialize in this procedure are not surprised to find patients from other states and even from abroad.

I recall one couple who came from a far distant country for donor insemination. For various personal reasons the wife could stay in New York for only one month, which meant that she would have to become pregnant during that cycle or abandon the plan entirely. Departing from my usual procedure of inseminating only once or twice according to the temperature graph, I decided on daily inseminations during her mid-cycle and did so until the temperature finally rose, indicating no more favorable days for insemination.

She left for home the next day, neither of us knowing whether she was at that moment pregnant or not. Three weeks later I received a letter with the heartwarming news that she had missed her period. Exactly which of those several inseminations was responsible for conception, no one will ever know, nor does it really matter.

Comparatively few people, however, can afford long-distance flights. For those who cannot, the distance to large cities can perhaps be bridged by semen "banks" containing frozen semen. There are already a great many normal babies conceived following insemination with frozen sperm from semen banks. The semen is stored for months at $-196°$ C in a liquid nitrogen refrigerator and thawed before use.

Some couples have a child by donor insemination and then, by an unexpected surprise, one of their own.

I have in mind a couple I'll call Nora and John, who came for donor insemination. The husband's sperm were consistently of very poor quality, despite various treatments that other doctors had prescribed. After agreeing that this was the best procedure for them, insemination with a donor was carried out and Nora became pregnant during her second cycle of treatment. She was delivered of a seven-and-a-half-pound baby boy, and everyone agreed that the baby "looks just like John."

Two and a half years later the couple returned in order to have another baby by the same procedure. Checking the husband's sperm, I found it to be as poor as ever. The first two cycles of insemination were unsuccessful, at which point the couple postponed further treatment, since they planned a vacation in Europe together. Imagine my surprise, as well as theirs, when Nora missed her period while on vacation. Upon her return, I confirmed the fact that she was pregnant. Out of curiosity I again checked John's sperm. The picture was about the same, for which anyone would have to conclude that the chances of conception were highly unlikely, though not impossible. A few months later I again delivered Nora, this time of a girl.

These events happened many years ago, but Nora has remained my patient and we have had an opportunity to discuss her family a number of times. I was impressed with the fact that they never seem to think of their children as different in any way and certainly appear to love them equally.

19

ADOPTION—PARENTHOOD FOR CHILDLESS COUPLES

. . . And a woman who held a babe against her bosom said: Speak to us of children. And he said: Your children are not your children. They are the sons and daughters of life's longing for itself. They come through you but not from you, and though they are with you, they belong not to you. You may give them your love but not your thoughts, for they have their own thoughts. You may house their bodies but not their souls, for their souls dwell in the house of tomorrow, which you cannot visit, not even in your dreams. You may strive to be like them, but seek not to make them like you. For life goes not backward nor tarries with yesterday. You are the bows from which your children as living arrows are set forth.

—KAHLIL GIBRAN, Lebanese mystic poet

To underscore these philosophic thoughts, I would like to point out a curious, almost universal phenomenon, which all obstetricians have noted. When a newborn baby is first seen by its own parents, there is a sheepish grin, a sort of "Did we produce that?" look of amazement. It is a perfectly natural feeling, a sort of comic awe. Every baby is tiny, helpless, like countless others; it could be any other baby, and the reaction would be much the same. There is as yet no real attachment, no true love.

This concept is terribly important for childless couples to realize, especially those who are destined to be unsuccessful in achieving the goal of pregnancy. Because the fact is, they might still have children, and the joys of parenthood are great even if they haven't physically borne the child.

Love for a child does not occur at the moment of birth. Love is a conditioned emotion developing gradually as the relationship slowly develops, as the parents feel needed, as the baby begins to respond, to recognize, to appreciate, to crawl under your skin! Such a relationship develops with an adopted child, or with a child born after donor insemination, in exactly the way it does with natural offspring. The joys of parenthood are undiminished. The gratifications, the rewards, are all the same.

I stress these points because there is a perfectly natural tendency for childless couples to despair if they are unsuccessful in achieving pregnancy. They may easily lose sight of the fact that it is not solely the "production" of the child that brings about the reciprocal love between parent and child; indeed, parents are usually unable to identify their own baby through a nursery window without a name tag. It is rather the caring for, the bringing up, the loving and the needing that bring about the unparalleled pleasures of parenthood.

Knowing this, I have always made it a policy to favor and support immediately any move on the part of childless couples to adopt. I point out that just *considering* adoption can bring a new and brighter outlook—at least it is an attempted step at something concrete. It does not mean that the couple need forego the possibility of having a child of their own as well. It does mean that parenthood is not postponed indefinitely.

Incidentally, it has long been a general impression that a childless couple has a greater chance of pregnancy after adopting a baby. The reason given is that the woman is no longer under the severe tension of waiting and wondering, finally relaxing enough to conceive. However, actual statistics have not borne out this conclusion. Yet the impression remains, probably explained by the fact that many women conceive after they *decide* to adopt, and then cancel plans for adoption. These cases are therefore not reflected in adoption statistics.

More important and interesting is the fact that parents who have both an adopted and a natural child confide that they love them equally. This holds true also for parents who have one child as a result of donor insemination and one of their own.

With this background in mind, one must realistically appraise adoption prospects as they exist today, compared with a decade or two ago.

Even in previous years, when there was a more plentiful supply of infants for adoption, the physician was first officially called up by the agency involved to supply information about the medical and emotional background of the applying couple.

Agencies and caseworkers would then follow up with interviews in an effort to determine the suitability of a particular couple. The social worker assigned would size up the family atmosphere of the potential parents, their age, health, emotional stability and, of course, their motivations in seeking a child. After completing the investigation (which could take a long time, because the demand has *always* been greater than the supply), the child might have been placed on a probationary basis. In final proceedings, the use of an attorney was important because the legalities governing adoption are so variable from state to state.

Today, although the same precautionary steps are taken by adoption agencies, there is one major difference. It is well known that currently there is a great scarcity of healthy infants (and even healthy toddlers) for adoption.

Several reasons account for this: the liberalization of abortion, the widespread availability of effective contraception and, most of all, changes in social mores which make it acceptable, and even fashionable, for an unwed mother to keep and raise her own child.

As a result, the majority of children available for adoption are so-called "hard to place" youngsters, meaning children who are already of school age, often from minority groups or mixed racial backgrounds, and children with emotional or physical handicaps. Although the special problems of children who have been in foster homes vary, it is reasonable to assume that there will be a delicate adjustment period during which the child, who may have doubts about his or her own worth, has some difficulty trusting new parents. Yet it is precisely the new adoptive parents who are able to give such children the chance to regain their self-confidence and to begin to dare to trust again, and finally to love. Actually, emphasis has been shifting from finding the "right child" for a family to finding the compatible "right family" for each child. Single, widowed or divorced individuals are no longer excluded as adoptive parents.

Realistically, however, most childless couples in America, who would ordinarily adopt from local agencies if enough children were available, are looking for an infant rather than an older child, and usually prefer one who has some degree of biological resemblance to them. Because of the frustrations due to the scarcity of adoptable children in this country, many such couples compromise by considering adoptions abroad. Indeed, foreign adoptions have increased greatly in recent years, involving countries such as South Korea, Southeast Asia and, more recently, South America. In all these instances, diplomatic, immigration, and legal policy issues were involved. In addition, there is the anxiety of the adoptive parents who may legitimately be concerned about the appearance and health of the baby.

But even foreign adoptions have been generally difficult, since most countries, particularly in Asia, prefer to care for their own children. Nevertheless, many prospective parents have been successful in such adoptive efforts if they were sufficiently motivated to investigate more fully.

HOW TO GO ABOUT IT

There are many agencies and organizations throughout the country which will give information and provide leads to those wishing to adopt children either in this country or abroad.

ADOPTION

For those wishing to adopt in the United States there are two large sources of information and assistance on the *national* level:

Children's Bureau
Department of Health, Education and Welfare
P.O. Box 1182
Washington, D.C. 20013

North American Center for Adoption
67 Irving Place
New York, New York 10003

(This is the parent organization of ARENA—Adoptive Resource Exchange of North America—and publishes newsletters and periodic reports about adoption availabilities. They will respond to inquiries with a list of agencies located in the prospective parents' own locality.)

In most large cities, there are also organizations composed of adoptive parents who wish to help others interested in adopting. Generally they can be found under such headings as the Council on Adoptable Children or The Adoptive Parents Association. Based on their own experience, these parent groups usually can provide personal information that is not otherwise obtainable and which can be extremely valuable to any couple seeking to adopt a child.

In the matter of international adoption, which is the increasing trend today, there are foreign-adoption parent-support groups, such as:

American Friends of Children (AFC)
110 Old Country Road
Deer Park, New York 11729

Adoptive Parents Committee (APC)
P.O. Box 306
Island Park, New York 11558

In addition, there are several parent groups actively involved in supplying necessary information, sources of foreign children, and general-support services to those prospective parents who wish to apply *directly:*

Latin American Parents Association (LAPA)
P.O. Box 72
Seaford, New York 11783

Families Interested in Adoption (FIA)
5543 Tonawanda Creek Road
North Tonawanda, New York 14120

Concerned Parents for Adoption (CPFA)
3 Marblestone Lane
Centereach, New York 11720

In writing to any of the parent groups, a stamped, self-addressed, legal-sized envelope should be enclosed, since they serve on a volunteer basis with very limited funds.

In addition to parent groups, there are specific Foreign Adoption Resource Agencies:

Foreign Adoption Center
Suite 202, 158 Filmore
Denver, Colorado 80206

Friends of Children, Inc., Conn.
14 Brookside Road
Darien, Connecticut 06820

Friends of Children, Inc., Georgia
4325 Memorial Dr., Suite 1
Decatur, Georgia 30032

Holt Adoption Program, Inc.
P.O. Box 288
Eugene, Oregon 97402

Project Orphans Abroad
4100 Franklin Blvd.
Cleveland, Ohio 44113

TDH Canada—Welcome A Child
53 Lakeshore Road
Pointe Claire
Quebec, Canada H98 4H4

Welcome House
P.O. Box 836
Doylestown, Pennsylvania 18901

World Family Adoptions
Rte. 1, 5048 Fairy Chasm Road
West Bend, Wisconsin 53095

On the State Level:
   In each state, the following agencies provide
applicants with information on adoption procedure
and referral to local agencies.

ALABAMA
Bureau of Child Welfare
Division of Adoption
Administrative Building
64 North Union Street
Montgomery, Alabama 36130

ALASKA
Department of Health and Social Services
Pouch HO5
Juneau, Alaska 99811

ARIZONA
Department of Economic Security
Child Welfare Department
3435 West Durango
Phoenix, Arizona 85009

ARKANSAS
Department of Social Welfare
Hendricks Hall
P.O. Box 1766
Little Rock, Arkansas 72203

CALIFORNIA
State Department of Health
Division of Adoptions and Foster Care
714/744 P Street
Sacramento, California 95814

COLORADO
Family and Children's Services
1575 Sherman Street
Denver, Colorado 80203

CONNECTICUT
Department of Children and Youth Services
Centralized Homefinding Unit
P.O. Box 902
Meriden, Connecticut 06450

DELAWARE
Children's Bureau
2005 Baynard Boulevard
Wilmington, Delaware 19802

DISTRICT OF COLUMBIA
Department of Human Resources
Adoption Division
122 C Street, N.W.
Washington, D.C. 20001

FLORIDA
Department of Social and Economic Services
Adoption Placement Unit
2030 Boulevard
Jacksonville, Florida 32201

GEORGIA
Department of Human Resources
State Placement Bureau
618 Ponce de Leon Avenue, N.E.
Atlanta, Georgia 30308

HAWAII
Department of Social Services
Public Welfare Division
1390 Miller Street
Honolulu, Hawaii 98809

IDAHO
Department of Health and Welfare
Statehouse
Boise, Idaho 83720

ILLINOIS
Department of Children and Family Services
INB Center
1 North Old State Capitol Plaza
Springfield, Illinois 62706

INDIANA
Division of Social Services
Child Welfare

141 S. Meridian Street (4th floor)
Indianapolis, Indiana 46225

IOWA
Division of Community Services
3619½ Douglas
Des Moines, Iowa 50310

KANSAS
State Department of Social Services
Division of Services to Children and Youth
State Office Building
Topeka, Kansas 66612

KENTUCKY
Department of Human Resources
Bureau of Social Services
275 East Main Street
Frankfort, Kentucky 40601

LOUISIANA
Department of Family Services
P.O. Box 44065
Baton Rouge, Louisiana 44065

MAINE
Department of Human Services
State House
Augusta, Maine 04333

MARYLAND
Department of Human Resources
Social Services Administration
11 South Street
Baltimore, Maryland 21202

MASSACHUSETTS
Department of Public Welfare

Social Services Division of Family and
Child Services
600 Washington Street
Boston, Massachusetts 02111

MICHIGAN
Department of Social Services
Adoption Division
300 South Capital Avenue
Lansing, Michigan 48926

MINNESOTA
Department of Public Welfare
Adoption Unit
Centennial Office Building
St. Paul, Minnesota 55155

MISSISSIPPI
Department of Public Welfare
Division of Social Services
2906 N. State Street
Jackson, Mississippi 30216

MISSOURI
Department of Welfare and Family Services
615 East 13 Street
Kansas City, Missouri 64104

MONTANA
Division of Social Services
Department of Public Welfare
Helena, Montana 59601

NEBRASKA
Department of Public Welfare
Division of Social Services
301 Centennial Mall South
Lincoln, Nebraska 68508

NEVADA
Department of Human Resources
Welfare Division
251 Jeanell Drive
Carson City, Nevada 89710

NEW HAMPSHIRE
Department of Health and Welfare
Bureau of Child and Family Services
8 Loudon Road
Concord, New Hampshire 03301

NEW JERSEY
Department of Human Services
Division of Youth and Family Services
1 South Montgomery Street
Trenton, New Jersey 08625

NEW MEXICO
Department of Social Services
Division of Adoption
P.O. Box 2348, Kennedy Hall
Santa Fe, New Mexico 87501,

NEW YORK
Department of Social Services
State Adoption Service, Room 850
Two World Trade Center
New York, New York 10047

NORTH CAROLINA
Department of Human Resources
Division of Social Services
325 N. Salisbury Street
Raleigh, North Carolina 27611

NORTH DAKOTA
Social Service Board of North Dakota

State Capitol Building
Bismarck, North Dakota 58505

OHIO
Adoption Resource Exchange
30 East Brond Street
Columbus, Ohio 43215

OKLAHOMA
Department of Institutions
Social and Rehabilitation Services
Division of Social Services
Sequoya Memorial Office Building
Oklahoma City, Oklahoma 73125

OREGON
Department of Human Resources
Children's Services Division
198 Commercial Street S.E.
Salem, Oregon 97310

PENNSYLVANIA
Department of Public Welfare
Bureau of Child Welfare
Health and Welfare Building
Harrisburg, Pennsylvania 17120

PUERTO RICO
Department of Social Services
Services to Families and Children
P.O. Box 11298
Fernandez Juncos Station
Santurce, Puerto Rico 00910

RHODE ISLAND
Department of Social and Rehabilitative Services
Family and Children's Services
610 Mt. Pleasant Avenue
Providence, Rhode Island 02908

SOUTH CAROLINA
(No centralized office)
Write to the Department of Social Services
in a particular county.

SOUTH DAKOTA
Department of Social Services
Office of Children, Youth and Family Services
State Office Building, Illinois Street
Pierre, South Dakota 57501

TENNESSEE
Department of Human Services
Division of Social Services
410 State Office Building
Nashville, Tennessee 37219

TEXAS
Department of Human Resources
John H. Reagan Building
Austin, Texas 78701

UTAH
Division of Family Services
150 West North Temple
Salt Lake City, Utah 84101

VERMONT
Department of Social and Rehabilitation Services
Human Services Agency
81 River Street
Montpelier, Vermont 05602

VIRGINIA
Department of Welfare
Division of Social Services
8007 Discovery Drive
Richmond, Virginia 23288

WASHINGTON
(No centralized office)
Write to Department of Social and Health
Services in a particular county.

WEST VIRGINIA
Department of Welfare
Division of Social Services
1900 Washington Street East
Charleston, West Virginia 25305

WISCONSIN
Department of Health and Social Services
Division of Community Services
State Office Building
1 West Wilson Street
Madison, Wisconsin 53702

WYOMING
Department of Public Assistance
Division of Social Services
Hathaway Building
Cheyenne, Wyoming 82002

The following books may be of additional help
to those contemplating adoption:

The Adoption Advisor by Joan McNamara. New
York: Hawthorne Books, Inc., 1975

The Adoption Dilemma. A Handbook for Adoptive Parents by Vincenette Scheppler. Rochester, New York: Arvin Publications, 1975.

Who Will Raise the Children? by James Levine.
New York: J.B. Lippincott, 1976.

For those interested specifically in resource
and reference information on foreign adoption:
Guide to Intercountry Adoptions. Available from

ODS—Massachusetts, 600 Washington St., Boston, Massachusetts 02111.

Handbook on Central and South American Adoption. Available from Project Orphans Abroad, 4100 Franklin Blvd., Cleveland, Ohio 44113.

Report on Foreign Adoptions. Available from Foreign Adoption Resources, 911 Cypress Drive, Boulder, Colorado 80303.

The Unbroken Circle, edited by Betty Kramer. Available from OURS INC., 3148 Humboldt Avenue South, Minneapolis, Minnesota 55408.

ACCEPTING CHILDLESSNESS

There is still another alternative for the infertile couple, which is to reexamine their goals. In many instances the "desire" to have a child is more motivated by parental or peer pressures than by the couple's own desires. (This is borne out most dramatically in those cases of psychogenic infertility where the woman, though appealing for help, actually prefers not to bear children.)

There is, in fact, a trend in this country to remain childless on purpose in order to achieve a freedom from responsibilities that would otherwise not be possible. Obviously those couples who share this view at the onset of their marriage will not seek help for infertility, but there are many other couples who at least harbor doubts regarding how much effort should be put into the "goal" of becoming parents. Those who have found medical testing too disagreeable and adoption too difficult often reassess their position, particularly if their frustrations are having eroding effects on their marriage. Rather than consider themselves "failures," they give up their quest for children and embark on a life of togetherness with a feeling of deep contentment in each other.

This does not mean that children are forever removed from their lives, for there are many possibilities of working with children through crafts or sports.

Although the trend toward remaining childless receives little support from organized religion, society, or the family unit, its advocates see it as a comfortable, acceptable alternative.

20

TEST-TUBE BIRTHS

For years, scientists have pondered the puzzling question of what to do for women who were infertile because of *hopelessly* blocked fallopian tubes, when this was considered the *only* reason for the infertility problem. If a normal egg, released each month, cannot enter at least one of the tubes, there could be no rendezvous with the sperm ascending from the other direction. Indeed, even the tiny sperm, no matter how actively motile, would be prevented from proceeding at whatever point the tubes were blocked. Nor did it matter whether the tubes were sealed because of pelvic disease, previous infection, sterilization, or pelvic surgery for other conditions—if the net result was bilateral complete closure with no prospect (or with failed attempts) to reopen them, conception was virtually impossible.

Of course, the standard treatment for blocked tubes has always been, *and continues to be,* some kind of surgical approach to unblock them. The promising new technique of microsurgery and special catheters has been discussed in Chapter

11. But even with these newer techniques, it is probable that if the tubes are sealed because of complete destruction of the lining (as happens in gonorrheal and other infections), the chances of conception and live births, even if they can be opened, are extremely slim. Similarly, women who have been sterilized by cautery (burning) of their tubes (rather than by plain tying and cutting) stand a very poor chance of effective recanalization by surgery. The prognosis is equally gloomy for those who have had multiple surgical attempts to correct blockage from any cause, since each attempt may cause further scarring. And, of course, for the woman with completely absent tubes it was quite hopeless. The thought of devising and implanting substitute, "artificial" tubes made of some tissue has been considered, but there have been no encouraging experiments to date.

For these reasons, it became evident that a different approach would have to be developed if a woman with hopelessly blocked or absent tubes was ever to bear a child. The logical question followed: what if her own egg and her husband's sperm could be fertilized *outside* the body (in vitro), then implanted into her uterus? Could it then not continue to grow and develop, just as it would have if fertilization had occurred normally in the tube, then been transported to the same location? Such an intriguing question had to be answered, even though the odds against it were formidable.

Several huge hurdles had to be overcome. It was already known from experimentation with animals that fertilization outside the body is a most complex process. Exacting nutrients would have to be found to simulate conditions existing in the body (which are still poorly understood). Then, once accomplished, the fertilized egg would have to reach a certain stage of development indicating at least a potential toward further growth. Finally, the most difficult, *how* and *when* to implant this tiny mass of cells into the womb?

It is known that in the human the fertilized egg takes several days to travel down the tube before implanting itself in the wall of the uterine cavity. If this was to be duplicated in vitro, then one would apparently have to wait several critical days before attempting implantation.

And then more questions: even if such a feat was possible and the embryo continued to grow in the woman's own womb, would all this tampering result in a fetal abnormality? At a time when almost every drug imaginable has been implicated as a possible cause of fetal harm, could such direct manipulations of the early developing cell mass be unaffected?

Somehow these questions had to be answered. Otherwise, countless women who had hopelessly blocked tubes could never bear a child of their own. Yes, the questions were important enough to investigate, much like a mystery.

In a way, the reader has already turned to the last chapter of this mystery novel and has learned the outcome—the successful birth of the Brown baby, the first "test-tube" baby, achieved in England by gynecologist Dr. Patrick Steptoe and his medical collaborator, physiologist Robert Edwards. But the chapters in between, leading up to this monumental climax, are also fascinating.

The history of attempts at fertilization outside the body is most intriguing.

The first report of such a fertilization was in 1936, made by Dr. Gregory Pincus of Harvard University, who united a *rabbit* egg and sperm in vitro (outside the body).

In 1944 Dr. John Rock, also from Harvard (he

and Dr. Pincus were pioneers in the development of contraceptive pills), claimed to have fertilized a *human* egg in vitro and watched it divide into several cells. Other scientists were of the opinion that the few cells observed were just parthenogenic cleavage (division of the egg without the involvement of sperm), probably induced by some incidental stimulation of the ovum.

Not until the mid 1960's did researchers know how to fertilize mammalian eggs outside the body on any regular basis. The basic groundwork was established by scientists in the United States and Britain, who solved the knotty problem of rabbit sperm "capacitation," a process that enabled the sperm to penetrate an egg in the laboratory.

Apparently sperm will not penetrate an egg unless "primed" (capacitated)—that is, the chemical inhibitors preventing the sperm from entering the egg must first be removed from the surface of the sperm. How this trick is accomplished in the body remains a mystery, but in the laboratory it is done by bathing the sperm in a special salt solution. In those early years, fertilization in vitro was confined to creatures no higher than rabbits, hamsters, and mice.

Meantime, back in England, Steptoe and Edwards continued their own cautious experiments for many years. Steptoe was a pioneer in the use of the laparoscope, and he worked on the mechanical technique of removing ova by the use of this slender telescopic instrument, combined with a suction needle. Edwards was developing special nutrients for fertilizing eggs so removed, as well as capacitating added sperm. Steptoe then worked out the mechanics of later returning the (dividing) fertilized eggs into the womb by a different process.

In 1970, Steptoe and Edwards reported in the

journal *Nature* that they had succeeded in observing fertilized *human* ova grow to the eight- and sixteen-cell stage. Several years later they began serious efforts to reimplant such test-tube ova, which are no larger than a dot.

They reported that, of some sixty attempted implants, only three showed any signs of lasting: two of these lasted but two weeks, and the third for nine weeks. These scientists postulated that their difficulties could be due to improper transferring of the eggs into the uterus, undetected chromosomal abnormalities, or interference with the acceptance of the fertilized egg by the very same hormones that were used to induce ovulation.

In 1974 there was a good bit of publicity about another English scientist who claimed to have implanted three fertilized embryos in women who subsequently gave birth, but he was either unwilling or unable to document his claims.

It was not until 1975 that Steptoe and Edwards produced their first definite "take"—but it turned out to be a misplaced implantation in the tube. It seemed that success was near, but yet very far.

The breakthrough came with recent research with rhesus monkeys, which provided the crucial clue that conventionally fertilized egg embryos as small as two cells might survive in the uterus. (Normally the human fertilized egg takes four or five days to reach the uterine cavity, and it was therefore considered necessary to keep an in-vitro egg that long before reimplanting.) On reflection, however, it is known that tubes that have been re-opened after disease or ligation can be considerably shortened, probably propelling a fertilized egg into the uterus much sooner than normally, and yet the egg survives and grows.

In any event, the monkey experiments convinced Steptoe and Edwards that an earlier implantation might work, and so the decision was made to reimplant at the eight-cell stage, or about two and a half days, which, incidentally, also reduced the complexities of sustaining the egg's development outside the body.

Thus the main difference between the historically successful experiment and the many previous failures was that, in prior cases, Steptoe and Edwards had tried to simulate the process as it occurs in the human body; normally, the egg multiplies to at least sixty-four or more cells before it reaches the womb for implantation. (As mentioned, however, the eggs of a woman with surgically shortened tubes may have a much shorter traveling time.)

The famous Brown baby was "conceived" on November 10, 1977, and then reimplanted two and a half days later.

In their earlier work, Drs. Steptoe and Edwards used various ovulation inducing drugs to obtain multiple eggs. More recently, and in the famous Brown case, the mother's natural ovulation was awaited by monitoring the pre-ovulatory phase of the cycle to determine the approximate time ovulation would occur. The next step, which was crucial, was to recognize the onset of the surge of pituitary luteinizing (L.H.) hormone by frequent urine samples—a key step in the recovery of a single ovum just prior to ovulation.

To locate the ovary, the laparoscope, a long telescopic optical instrument, is inserted through a small abdominal incision to see the exact area from which the mature egg or eggs have ripened. Under direct vision a separate aspirating needle is inserted into the ovaries to draw out the egg itself. The extracted egg is transferred to a culture dish containing serum and nutrients. To this is added sperm from the husband, previously processed to capacitate (prime) them.

Once an egg has been fertilized by one of the many spermatozoa, it is then transferred to another dish of sustaining nutrients, and its development to a several-cell stage (blastocyst) is observed. The woman meanwhile is receiving further hormonal treatment to prepare her uterine lining. The embryo is monitored in its divisions until after about fifty hours it reaches the eight-cell stage.

The developing cluster of cells is then transferred by means of a thin catheter into the cervix. The embryo itself, carried in a smaller cannula within the catheter, is placed near the uterine wall, so that it can implant itself in the body of the uterus.

After the transfer is made, the cannula must be reexamined under the microscope to see if the embryo is gone, since it is too small to be seen with the naked eye. It appeared, too, that implantation was more likely to be successful if it were performed in the evening, due to an apparent diurnal variation in hormone levels. In any event, once the embryo was implanted, the pregnancy was carefully monitored. This was done by ultrasound, amniocentesis at 16 weeks, and placental function tests to rule out any genetic abnormalities prior to birth.

The rest is truly living history!

To the medical researcher or practicing clinician, the remarkable birth of the first "test-tube" baby immediately calls attention to two things: first, that couples will obviously go to extraordinary lengths to achieve a much-wanted pregnancy; second, that much more research must be done along the lines of *preventing or curing the*

*type of tubal disorders that have led to the neces-
sity for such a complex, roundabout procedure as*
fertilization in vitro.

It is estimated that from 20 to 50 percent of
childless women have *some* degree of tubal problem; the average would be about 35 percent for all
infertile women.

Surgery for tubal disease has been briefly discussed on p. 85, including the development of the
newer technique of microsurgery. In addition,
there is ongoing research at Lenox Hill Hospital
in New York City with new, delicate, elongated
"balloon" catheters for dilating diseased *coronary
arteries*, which I feel can be equally effective in
many cases of diseased fallopian tubes. I contem-
plate using this new "tube-shaped" balloon in infertility surgery at the same institution, and it
appears to have exciting potential in dilating fallopian tubes more naturally than the spherical
balloon catheters that I have used for many years.
As with other procedures for tubal disorders, this
novel approach would, of course, have to be
judged in terms of pregnancies achieved.

Obviously, any significant breakthrough or improvement in conventional (or unconventional)
methods of treating tubal disorders *that would
lead to a significantly higher live birth rate than
we now have* would accomplish the goal in a more
natural way.

Pending such developments, however, the
achievement of a live birth by bypassing the tubes
by fertilization outside the body must be heralded
as nothing short of spectacular.

One may well ask why there has been no significant research on in-vitro human fertilization for
infertility in our own country. There are several
reasons. One is that, normally, researchers start
testing new medical procedures on animals, such

as rabbits or mice, then on nonhuman primates, such as monkeys or apes, before experimenting with humans. We do not have full-term primate births to pave the way.

Furthermore, the legality of this controversial process (and in particular the legal status of fertilized eggs before implantation) needs clarification in this country, where lawsuits are commonplace for any procedure that significantly deviates from the "tried and true" or "approved." But approved by whom?

Far from gaining approval in this country, federal support for research on human in-vitro fertilization was halted in 1975. A new National Ethics Advisory Board was established in January, 1978, which rules on all human experimentation and controls research in any institution receiving federal funding for any of its activities. Specific research proposals are being reviewed and will be recommended on an individual-case basis. One proposal to be considered involves experimentation with in-vitro fertilized *animal* eggs exposed to various drugs and toxins, to detect their possible influence on birth defects (which may appear later in life). A reason for this concern is that normally only the strongest sperm reach the egg for fertilization in the body, whereas in the test tube, both strong and weak sperm may have almost equal access.

There is also the fear that, although the Brown case was apparently completely successful, other test-tube babies might be born with mental or physical defects. One can envision lawsuits by such children against the physicians who "created" them, or even against their own parents.

The question of the legal status of fertilized eggs before implantation is in itself intriguing, if we keep in mind the fact that in the human body the majority of actual conceptions never progress to term; many are aborted so "silently" that the mother may not even have been aware that she was pregnant. This would hardly be called a "bedroom experiment," but those are the facts.

From the medical point of view, it should also be noted that even if test-tube fertilization were "approved," many infertile women are really unsuitable candidates. That is, aside from hopelessly blocked tubes (the prime indication), there may be weakness of the sperm (not uncommon), poor ovulatory function, or some malformation of the uterus, making it unlikely that implantation by any means will result in proper growth. Dr. Edwards himself estimates that such a special procedure would at best be helpful in only about seventeen percent of applicants with tubal problems.

There are other far-reaching ramifications. According to Steptoe and Edwards, the freezing and storing of embryos (already a routine in cattle) could provide an *infertile* woman with a whole family of children after a single procedure in which a number of eggs are obtained. Hormones would be used to stimulate multiple production of eggs. The eggs would then be surgically removed and exposed to the husband's sperm, then cultured briefly in the laboratory.

Thus far the procedure is similar to what has already been accomplished. The next step, however, has never been done in humans as far as is known. The fertilized egg cells that show signs of normal embryonic development could be frozen. This would provide enough time before future implantation to screen the embryo for any genetic defects. Then, at intervals of a year or more, the embryos could be implanted (one by one) in the woman's uterus and allowed to mature into babies in the normal manner.

As expected, the birth of the first test-tube baby touched off debates about the ethical, moral and religious considerations involved. As one theologian put it, he could foresee "designing our descendants . . . fabricating the next generation . . . making reproduction synonymous with manufacturing. . . ." Others saw it as an ethical nightmare, with a change from doctoring the patient to doctoring the human race, and still others were equating "destruction" of apparently live embryos with abortion of far more developed fetuses within the body. Still others could foresee the possibility of implanting a fertilized egg in a third party, who would act as a surrogate mother, giving up the child after birth. "The rich may hire the poor to bear their children for them," it was pointed out, or else could "buy" embryos from someone whose genetic background they particularly like. The ramifications are endless.

It should perhaps be noted here for clarification that the type of surrogate mother envisioned would ostensibly be implanted with an egg already fertilized outside the body; the source of the egg and sperm for the parents-to-be would ostensibly come from them, but could also be "donated" by others.

This is not the same as the "parent by proxy" surrogate mother, who has already made headlines in this country. In these instances of "wombs for rent," men have arranged for women to be impregnated with their sperm (their own wives being infertile), then adopting the child. In one Michigan case, the infertile wife herself inseminated the surrogate mother, who became pregnant as a result. Said the attorney involved, "Michigan physicians wouldn't touch the situation because of the malpractice threat." However, he also pointed out some obvious dilemmas raised by surrogate motherhood; for instance: what if the proxy mother decides to keep the child? How would the courts rule? To say the least, it would be an extraordinary situation.

Therefore, the present debates concern not the above situation but rather the more bizarre speculation about the creation of superbeings and a general image of an Aldous Huxley vision of embryos that are bred en masse in artificial wombs.

Nor should the process of in-vitro fertilization be confused with "cloning." Unlike test-tube fertilization, which actually lets nature take its course (sperm from the father and an egg from the mother unite, although in a dish), cloning is asexual, single-parent reproduction. In other words, cloning is not a mixture of genes from two parents but is a genetic copy of a single parent. It is based on the astonishing fact that virtually every cell in any organism (vegetable, animal, plant, bacterium, human) carries *all* the genetic information needed to create the whole organism. In a sense, every cell of the body with a nucleus is a potential individual. Most experiments to date have been on the nuclei of frog cells and tadpoles. For example, when the nucleus is taken from the skin cell of a frog and placed in the egg of another frog whose nucleus has been removed, that egg can develop into a twin of the skin-cell donor.

It has been found, however, that the nuclei of adult mammalian cells are generally poor cloning material, possibly because their genes have been irreversibly "turned off." Because of the relatively small size of such cells, the difficulties in manipulation, and the fact that they must eventually develop in a womb, most scientists agree that human cloning is not only impractical but that it realistically presents completely unsolvable ethical and social problems. Dr. Edwards himself saw little prospects for cloning except in agriculture.

Although the concepts of test-tube babies and surrogate mothers are thought-provoking and dramatic, they are not really new and have been considered for many years. In one of my own previous publications (1970), I wrote:

> In these days of heart and other organ transplants, there are also some dramatic future possibilities in the field of infertility. For example, if a woman can conceive but has tubes blocked in such a way that a fertilized egg cannot pass into the uterus, the doctor may be able to remove the egg from the tube and implant it into the patient's own uterus. In other cases, where the tubes are hopelessly blocked, it may be possible to remove the woman's ovum, fertilize it in a laboratory with sperm provided by the husband, then reimplant it in her womb. Some embryologists have suggested a much more startling and controversial concept, that of "host mothers" being paid to give birth to babies conceived in test tubes from the eggs of women unable to bear children themselves.
>
> An artificial placenta may not be far away either. National Heart Institute researchers have shown that an artificial tank of vital fluids plus an artificial lung can "mother" a lamb fetus for several days. This raises the possibility that human fetuses in distress might be removed from the womb and grown to term in such an environment, and that premature infants can thus be eased through crises that now overwhelm them.

Much has come to pass. Animal researchers are slowly moving toward a *true* test-tube birth. In one experiment, scientists from the United States and Canada preserved lambs withdrawn prematurely from their mothers. Kept in plastic bags that contained a solution similar to amniotic fluid, the fetal lambs were then linked to a mechanical blood-circulating device. After surviving for varying periods of time in this environment, they were then "reborn."

Other researchers have kept mice embryos alive outside the body for over eight days. Although this does not sound like a long time, it actually represents almost half of the full gestational period for a mouse.

The idea that scientists will ever be able actually to produce artificial wombs that will accept test-tube humans from conception to birth sounds like pure science fiction, but then so did many of the achievements already accomplished.

Nevertheless, the unraveling of the mysteries of reproduction appears to be moving at an astonishing speed. Recently, scientists involved with DNA and genetic technology, working in various parts of the world, reported the identification of a *single gene* among the millions in a single human cell: The gene discovered directs the production of hemoglobin (the iron compound that carries oxygen to the blood). Doctors can now determine from samples of fluid surrounding the human fetus whether the fetus suffers from certain forms of anemia, by detecting the presence or absence of that particular gene. Detection previously required a sample of fetal blood, which is much more risky. Though this type of anemia is rare, researchers are predicting that within a few years they will have the genetic code to many more common disorders, such as cystic fibrosis, for example.

Surrogate mothers, cloning, and genes aside, let us now return to the work of Steptoe and Edwards, and the sensational achievement of the first test-tube birth.

The term *"test-tube baby"* may itself be somewhat confusing or misleading, since this same term has been previously applied to several other procedures.

One is the common instance where infertility is due to complete *male* sterility (no sperm, or almost none), in which the wife elects to undergo therapeutic ("artificial") insemination of donor sperm for the purpose of making her pregnant. This has been a time-honored and recognized therapeutic procedure for many decades and is described in detail (AID) in Chapter 18.

Another procedure is similar, but uses the husband's own sperm when there is inherent weakness of the sperm or difficulty with ascent into the womb. This is called therapeutic (again "artificial") insemination with the husband's sperm (AIH), and is described on pp. 46–47 and 56–57.

In a sense, then, the procedure used for the birth of *the first test-tube baby is but one step beyond what is being done today, when infertility requires therapeutic insemination of the husband's sperm*. The breakthrough by Steptoe and Edwards involved the first successful birth after fertilizing the human ovum *outside* the body, with reimplantation into the womb. (Obviously, therapeutic husband insemination does not work if the tubes are blocked, since there will be no access to the egg.)

It seems to me that the ethical and moral questions raised avoid the central issue, which is that the first test-tube birth is simply a further scientific attempt to help a previously hopeless childless couple become parents when medical circumstances prevented them from doing so naturally. No artificial egg or sperm were either discovered or used. And it is not "making babies in glass dishes instead of beds"; its only application is when making babies in bed is impossible. A spokesman for the American Medical Association saw no ethical problem, since the procedure is simply an extension of artificial insemination and sperm banks, which we have had for years. Steptoe himself has stated that he saw no ethical problem. "We are not creating life . . . we have merely done what many people try to do in all kinds of medicine—to help nature. . . ." And though the widespread use of the procedure is certainly not just around the corner, the Brown case has nevertheless given countless women new hope.

It would also seem to me that human intervention is hardly unethical when it seeks to correct nature's defects. Medical practice has played this very role from the beginning. The procedure at every point attempted to simulate nature, in the absence of functioning fallopian tubes. And it succeeded.

There will always be differing concepts of ethical conduct, and often reversal when reality of experience proves them to be in error. In my thirty years of clinical practice, I am reminded that similar grave misgivings prevailed concerning therapeutic donor insemination; yet the couples involved have proved to be the happiest of parents. But even today, donor insemination stands where contraception stood about sixty years ago. In fact, *any* innovative procedure related to reproduction, such as the test-tube baby, is destined to be controversial. It lies in the field of sex.

Any change in custom or practice in this emotionally charged area of sex and reproduction is apt to elicit a response from established custom and law of concerned negation at first, then negation with less concern, then gradual curiosity, study, evaluation, and finally a very slow but steady acceptance by the majority.

Naturally there will be more research and study. But there is no question but that in-vitro fertilization represents a major advance, with the promise of still more breakthroughs in embryo research, a better understanding of birth defects and their prevention, and a notable milestone in the treatment of infertility.

There can be no progress without some risk as well. Since I deal primarily with infertility problems, I am personally delighted with the spectacular achievement of Steptoe and Edwards. I believe that, in time, it will be looked upon as the pioneer work of the "past" that has brought new hope and *new life* to many otherwise infertile couples.

21

PREVENTION OF INFERTILITY

Some of the main reasons why infertility is on the increase have already been mentioned: the rise in venereal disease, certain contraceptives such as the pill and the IUD, abortions, and the postponement of marriage until less fertile years. Any measures that diminish these factors will, of course, be helpful in halting or at least decreasing the sharp rise in infertility problems that specialists are seeing today. It is largely a matter of education and the correction of misinformation, and the medical profession has a responsibility in both areas.

It might also be noted that the subject of infertility is an almost totally neglected area in school programs. The only time it may come up is perhaps to scare youngsters when discussing the ominous consequences of venereal disease in health or hygiene classes.

Since it is well known that many young people are sexually active, it would be more helpful to point out some pertinent facts. Gonorrhea, for example, is without obvious symptoms in about 80 percent of women who have it. If a female is sexually active, particularly with multiple partners, her best protection is the use of a condom. In addition, a pelvic examination and cultures for gonorrhea every few months might disclose the disease even when unexpected.

Symptoms that both men and women should be aware of include any unusual discharge from the penis or vagina, any open sores near the genitals, and pain on urination. It is important to stress that both gonorrhea and syphilis are *curable* diseases if diagnosed and treated promptly. In my own practice I see fair numbers of women of all ages who express a specific fear about the presence of venereal disease. Some are adolescents or young unmarried women with multiple partners, some are married women who have a legitimate concern, either because of their own indiscretions or those of their husbands, some are call girls who require tests with repeated regularity, and some are middle-aged women who are worried because of an unexpected fling. Whatever the circumstance, it is reassurance that is asked for.

Among contraceptive measures, the condom is the only one that will protect against pregnancy and most cases of venereal disease simultaneously. Unfortunately, it is not always the preferred method. The diaphragm is an excellent, harmless method of preventing pregnancy, but not venereal disease. However, the diaphragm will in no way interfere with future fertility.

The contraceptive pill, on the other hand, must always be considered with caution. Considering only the fertility aspects, it should be noted that a woman is ill advised to use the pill to "regulate" menstrual cycles that have either not established themselves with regularity, or are consistently irregular. Such women already show evidence of faulty or absent ovulatory function, and the prolonged use of the pill will further suppress their hormonal function. It is the woman with irregular menstrual cycles who is most apt to encounter a complete ovulatory shutdown after the pill has been discontinued. Though this is not harmful to her health, it is a keen disappointment if she wishes to become pregnant. This is one reason why women who plan to have a family at *any* time in the future should take a "breather" from the pill every year or two to see if spontaneous periods recur. If not, it is well to know it before they are ready to conceive.

The choice of an intrauterine device should also be made with care. The popularity of the method is quite understandable; it gives a high degree of protection, permits complete spontaneity, and has none of the systemic side effects of the pill. However, the IUD is not for everyone who requests it. Women with heavy or painful periods are likely to have these symptoms aggravated, and women who have had any previous history of pelvic inflammatory disease (PID) are prime candidates for a "lighting up" of a possibly smoldering infection, with dire consequences regarding future fertility. The IUD has also been implicated in increased risk of pelvic inflammation in women without such a definite history. This may be quite mild and readily curable with antibiotics. Large-scale statistics indicate that the vast majority of women who use IUD's notice a prompt return of their fertility after its removal.

Women with an unwanted pregnancy who plan to have an abortion should be sure that it is done by someone they trust to be highly competent. Should they develop any symptoms or signs of postabortal infection (fever, pain, foul discharge), they should report it without delay, so that proper antibiotic measures can be started at once.

Women who plan to start their family when in their mid-thirties should be aware that fertility normally gradually decreases with age. Furthermore, if there should be an infertility problem, there will be less time (and more urgency) to solve it.

22

PRESELECTING
YOUR BABY'S SEX?

"It's a boy!"—or—"It's a girl!" are usually the first words to greet a new parent. The standard reply is: "As long as it's healthy!"

Years ago not much thought was given to *pre*selecting the baby's sex before conception, since it was always considered pretty much a fifty-fifty proposition anyway, even when the odds seemed unkind.

I am reminded of a husband of a patient whom I was about to deliver. Already the father of three sons, he had been sweating it out in the waiting room. I finally brought him the news—another fine, healthy boy. He gave a faint smile of relief that the delivery was over, but his disappointment was also evident, and I commented at it with obvious sympathy and understanding. "No matter," he said with a sigh, "it was my second choice, anyway!"

Can there actually be a choice, or at least a way of significantly shifting the odds? Since there have been several books and articles on "choos-

171

ing" the sex of your baby, some clarification seems in order.

Several different methods have been advocated over the years, in an attempt to predetermine a baby's sex before conception. The one best known to the public has to do with coital timing. At best, it can be summarized as inconclusive and contradictory, but here are the facts:

About twenty-five years ago, the late Dr. Sophia Kleegman noted that artificial insemination just before or at the time of ovulation produced a 70-to-80-percent male offspring, whereas insemination two or more days before ovulation produced a majority of females.

Dr. Landrum B. Shettles not only agreed with Kleegman's observations but claimed to have identified two distinct sperm types under the phase-contrast microscope. He believed that sperm with small heads carried the Y (boy) chromosome, whereas those with large heads carried the X (girl) chromosome. He then hypothesized that the smaller male sperm traveled faster and would reach the egg first at the optimal (ovulation) time, when cervical alkalinity is highest. The slower but stronger female sperm, he postulated, do better two or more days prior to ovulation and thrive better in an acid environment. He therefore advised, for a male child, abstinence until ovulation time, then intercourse preceded by an alkaline (baking-soda) douche, with deep penetration of the penis (preferably from the rear) to help ensure deposition of sperm near the cervix. To beget a female child, he advised intercourse two to three days before ovulation (no prior abstinence required), preceded by an acid (vinegar or acetic acid) douche, with shallow penile penetration by the husband in a face-to-face position. The theory was that coitus on the day of ovulation favors male offspring, since male sperm are likely to reach the egg before the slower female sperm. Coitus two or three days before ovulation favors a female baby, since most male sperm will have died off before ovulation.

Meantime, back in Chicago, Dr. Melvin Cohen, attempting to duplicate Kleegman's observations in a large series of insemination cases, could not corroborate her findings; nor could he corroborate Shettles' emphasis on cervical mucus, since he found no correlation between quality of mucus at insemination and the sex of the baby.

Shettles' microscopic observations were also strongly disputed by several other scientists, who felt that he was looking at optical distortions.

It remained for Dr. Rodrigo V. Guerrero to provide further clues to this apparent impasse, as well as an additional haze. In studying large series in which there was *natural* intercourse (not insemination) at the time of ovulation, he found a slightly higher percentage of girls, which appeared to contradict Shettles' findings. In the *artificially inseminated* group the probability of males did rise slightly (approximately 60 percent), but far less than predicted by either Kleegman or Shettles. Using temperature graphs, the picture was further confused by the question of exactly when Guerrero considered the time of ovulation to be (the graph is not a precise test). In any event, it appeared that predictions of the baby's sex might be completely different when fertilization was by insemination rather than natural.

Two books for the general public were published in 1977. One, *Choose Your Baby's Sex*, was by Shettles, in which he continued to advocate exposure during ovulation to conceive boy babies and away from ovulation for girls. The other, *Boy or Girl?*, was by Elizabeth M. Whelan, a research associate at Harvard, who took exactly the opposite stand. From her own surveys Whelan assured readers that *girl* babies are conceived at the time of ovulation and boy babies several days before! It would seem that the two books together might convince readers (even better than a physician's skepticism) that our knowledge of sex selection is at best highly speculative.

A completely different approach to preselect the sex of offspring is by separating X (girl) and Y (boy) sperm. This has been attempted in many complex ways, such as by electrical surface charge, the use of antisera, mechanical centrifugation, staining for fluorescence, and exposure to different pH (acid/alkaline) media, the latter, incidentally, giving results contrary to Shettles' theory.

The most interesting research has been reported by Dr. Ronald Ericsson, a reproductive physiologist, who has managed to separate X and Y sperm by an ingenious method. He conducts a "race" where the sperm swim through a glass column through increasingly dense layers of albumin (a natural fluid found in blood plasma). The faster male sperm (Y) get to the finish line first and by repeating the process Ericsson was able to get a concentration of about 90 percent male sperm. These, administered by insemination, would be expected to produce a great preponderance of boy babies.

So far the number of cases have been too few and the time interval too short to form conclusions; it may take another year or so to see if the statistics are as predicted. Of course, this process won't help the couple that wants a girl, nor will it please patients who prefer not to go through the procedure of insemination or a sperm bank.

Since the method also weeds out weak sperm, however, it may have an additional application in enhancing male fertility. In cases where the sperm are subnormal, the yield of Y (boy) sperm is expectedly lower than in normal specimens.

If any method of preselection of sex were easily possible, it would undoubtedly have profound social and genetic consequences. Most surveys indicate no particular preference except in the birth *order*, a boy being preferred first. Ericsson's method would also lead in that direction. After a number of years, a preponderance of males could have a significant sociological effect. According to Columbia University sociologist Amitai Etzioni, it might lead to "a society with some of the rougher features of a frontier town." A country with many more men may mean higher crime rates (since men account for the bulk of criminal statistics), an increase in prostitution because of the scarcity of women, an increase in homosexuality, and more tension between races and classes.

Perhaps it's for the best that at the present time the ratio is still about fifty-fifty.

Although we do not now have a completely reliable method of preselecting a baby's sex, there is one 100 percent method of knowing whether it's a boy or girl *after* conception. This involves amniocentesis, the withdrawal of amniotic fluid at about sixteen weeks of gestation, and a study of the cells thus obtained. Such information, however, is usually an incidental finding when amniocentesis is done for the purpose of detecting fetal abnormalities. In many such cases the parents specifically ask *not* to be told the sex of the baby so early, in order that they may have the pleasure of being surprised at delivery.

Part Four

SEX AND THE BIOLOGY OF REPRODUCTION

23

SEX ANATOMY

External female anatomy is exceedingly well appreciated by both sexes. But when it comes to the internal organs of reproduction, it appears that most women do not understand the structure or workings of their own bodies.

The vagina is an elastic sheathlike canal about four to five inches long. It expands very easily to accommodate, at various times, a tampon during menstruation, a penis during intercourse, and a baby's head during delivery.

The walls of the vagina continually produce a cleansing and lubricating film of moisture, making it a self-cleansing organ. Near the vaginal entrance are two small glands (named Bartholin's) that produce an additional lubricant, mainly on sexual stimulation.

The uterus (womb; belly in Latin) is the size and shape of a small pear. It is hard and muscular and measures only two and a half to three inches in total length.

During pregnancy the uterus expands tremendously, up to forty times its normal size. This is possibly because of the many elastic fibers meshed with the powerful muscle fibers, the same muscles that play such an important role in the contractions of labor and delivery.

The inner lining of the uterus is triangular, soft and smooth, and is called the endometrium (Greek for "within the womb"). The uterine openings of the fallopian tubes enter the womb at the top.

The lower portion of the uterine cavity is very narrow and is called the cervical canal. It is surrounded by the cervix (Latin for "neck"), the external opening of the uterus. About half of the cervix actually projects into the vagina and can be felt as a firm protrusion. The cervix can be visually examined by the doctor, and it is this organ which is the principal target of "Pap" cancer-prevention smears.

The opening in the cervix is very narrow, and this tight passage serves to keep the inside of the uterus free of germs. The cervical opening is the first passageway through which sperm must pass.

The tubes (oviducts; "egg ducts") are also known as fallopian tubes after the sixteenth-century physician Gabriello Fallopio, who mistakenly thought they were "ventilators" for the womb. Each is about four inches long, rather slender and delicate.

The tubes afford a passageway for the eggs to reach the cavity of the womb. Actually, the tubes are not directly connected to the ovaries but have a funnel-like opening near the corresponding ovary with delicate fringes capable of moving toward the ovary and receiving an egg.

The inner passage of the tube has a velvety lining containing brushlike hairs called cilia, which move in the direction of the womb. The actual passageway is no wider than the lead in a pencil.

The ovaries (from the Latin *ova*, meaning eggs) are two in number, lying near the sides of the uterus. The ovaries produce the egg cells (ova), potentially about half a million, but actually only one a month during a woman's reproductive life, or some four hundred in all. Each ovary is about the size of a flattened robin's egg.

About three hundred years ago a Dutch physician named De Graaf first linked the ovaries to reproduction. He suggested the name ovary because he assumed (incorrectly) that an ovarian follicle, which houses a potentially developing egg, corresponds to a bird's nest. In any event, the human egg follicle that matures each month of reproductive life is known as a Graafian follicle. Ovaries are also called "gonads" from the Greek *gone*, which means seed.

24

THE MENSTRUAL CYCLE

Every woman knows that a missed menstrual period is often associated with pregnancy. She also knows that if she gets her period, there is virtual certainty of no pregnancy. The onset of a menstrual flow, particularly a "late" one, is thus greeted with elation if she does not want to be pregnant, or with keen disappointment if she does. Menstruation becomes the first familiar and overt sign associated with reproduction.

It wasn't always so. Long ago the relationship between menstruation and reproduction was not understood. In fact, scientists once thought that a woman's most fertile time was during her period.

Today we know that menstruation is but one phase of the reproductive cycle, a cycle of hormonal interaction so complex that any deviation can easily interfere with fertility. It is precisely our increased understanding of what occurs in the various organs of the body that has made possible the many advances in the treatment of menstrual disorders and infertility.

Menstruation (from the Latin *mensis,* meaning month) refers to the monthly shedding of the uterine lining. It is the only time when blood is not associated with injury, but rather with health.

Menstruation makes way for a new uterine lining. At the time the old lining is shed, it is almost twice as thick as it was after the last menstrual period. Thus each month the lining (endometrium) is renewed, revitalized and rebuilt for a specific purpose=the reception of a fertilized egg. All this is accomplished mainly by the feverish activity of the two female hormones, estrogen and progesterone. Many women insist that their menstrual cycles are regular as clockwork, but this is not borne out when careful records are kept.

Every woman is *normally* irregular at the beginning and at the end of her reproductive years. When periods first start in the teens (called menarche) they are characteristically irregular, and the same thing happens when a woman approaches menopause. The reason is that when a woman first starts menstruating, she lacks the regularizing action of progesterone, produced only by ovulation (egg release). Ovulation begins to falter near menopause, which accounts for the irregularity again at that time of life.

By the same token, lack of ovulation also means lack of fertility. So both the young girl and the older woman usually have a number of infertile cycles, attributable to the same capricious inactivity of the glands. Notice that I said "usually." This accounts for the occasional youngster who gets pregnant at age fourteen, as well as the occasional woman of forty-six who has a "menopause baby."

Actually, the number of high school girls who do become pregnant is a sad reminder that fertility does begin somewhere in the teens, and this fertility can extend until menopause, the end of menstrual and reproductive life. With an average age span of seventy-five, a woman thus spends the last third of her life in an infertile state (unlike animals, whose reproductive capacity lasts through their life span).

While this capacity to bear children is usually taken for granted, there is a lot of behind-the-scenes activity going on in various glands and organs concerned with reproduction.

The menstrual cycle is caused by and controlled by the activity of four hormones, two from the pituitary gland at the base of the skull and two from the ovaries.

The stage is set by the pituitary, the so-called "master gland." The pituitary is controlled by a higher center called the hypothalamus or midbrain, the seat of emotions. This explains why and how the emotions can influence glandular function.

In any event, triggered by the hypothalamus, the pituitary starts to secrete its follicle-stimulating hormone, whose function is, not surprisingly, to stimulate the follicles in the ovaries. Follicles are minute sacs containing unripe eggs. This follicle-stimulating hormone (FSH) zeros in on one particular follicle. In response, this target follicle begins to mature and the egg sac begins to secrete a hormone, estrogen. Estrogen is the chief female sex hormone and has a multitude of important functions throughout life. But in this particular context its role is to cause a thickening of the lining of the womb. This is the first step in preparing for a fertilized egg.

With the rise in level of estrogen production, the pituitary now begins to secrete another hormone called luteinizing hormone (LH). Now this hormone zeros in on the same ovarian follicle, stimulating it to release the mature egg. When the egg is released, the process is called ovulation.

Ovulation occurs approximately halfway between menstrual periods in a twenty-eight-day cycle, but is subject to change according to the delicate daily hormonal balance and other variables.

As the level of luteinizing hormone increases, the now empty follicle undergoes a startling change in color to orange-yellow and is now called a "corpus luteum" (yellow body). In its new form it produces not only estrogen but a new hormone called progesterone. Progesterone (literally "for gestation") causes the uterine lining to thicken even more to prepare a soft bed in case an egg becomes fertilized.

If there is no pregnancy, the pituitary (always reacting to the hypothalamus) ceases its production of luteinizing hormone, and the corpus luteum begins to wither.

As it shrinks, its production of progesterone and estrogen declines, at first gradually, then more sharply; it is this "withdrawal" from the bloodstream of estrogen and progesterone that actually triggers menstruation. The same mechanism is in play when birth-control pills (which contain similar hormones) are stopped after a certain number of days; a "period" follows.

With the menstrual flow, the uterine lining is shed. This is often described as the "bloody tears of a disappointed uterus." The woman knows she is not pregnant. The old cycle is over and a new cycle is about to begin. Each new cycle is initiated by the pituitary gland in the same way, and this process is repeated month after month for some twenty-five to thirty years, unless pregnancy intervenes.

If pregnancy does take place, there's a lot of new activity. The fertilized egg produces a very special hormone called chorionic gonadotropin, which comes to the rescue of the corpus luteum (empty egg sac) just as the latter is about to wither from the withdrawal of pituitary support. Instead, with this new support of chorionic gonadotropin, the corpus luteum continues to function, producing estrogen and progesterone in even greater quantities. Since there is no drop in the secretion of these two hormones, there is no signal for the pituitary to stimulate any more follicles. The woman is pregnant, and both ovulation and menstruation are suspended for the entire course of the pregnancy.

However, the corpus luteum cannot supply the needed estrogen and progesterone indefinitely. It is already overworked. But nature has taken care of that, too. A few weeks after conception, the cells of the embryonic afterbirth (placenta) take over the function of producing these hormones and continue to do so right up to the time of delivery.

Thus it can be said that the main organs concerned with menstruation are the ovaries, uterus and pituitary (with the hypothalamus ruling in the background). For smooth functioning, however, it is also important for two other glands to cooperate: the thyroid, located in the neck, and the adrenals, atop each kidney. They, too, can influence menstruation and fertility. Their role must also be assessed in any complete investigation of infertility.

25

THE REPRODUCTIVE
PROCESS

Conception is the most miraculous process in biology, and nature has cleverly seen to it that reproduction will continue by making sexual intercourse so pleasurable. Here is the physiological explanation of the way it happens.

The female ovum is the largest single human cell but is actually only 1/200 of an inch in diameter, which is smaller than the tiniest grain of sand. It is relatively large because it contains a store of nutrients to sustain a growing embryo during the few days' journey until it is embedded in the wall of the womb. The egg itself has no means of mobility and must depend upon physiological factors (and luck) to be "picked up" by the open end of the fallopian tube and then slowly be propelled toward the uterus by hairlike cilia in the wall of the tube.

Actually, the egg can survive for only about two days. If it is not fertilized within that time it will gradually disintegrate, wherever it happens to be located.

Not all eggs released by the ovaries are fit for reproduction. At least 15 percent cannot be fertilized, and an additional 25 percent which *are* fertilized die before, or soon after, implantation in the uterus. In many cases, resorption takes place without the woman's being aware that she was pregnant. Such early death of eggs and embryos is a universal phenomenon among all animal species.

The follicle or sac from which the ovum is extruded is relatively large because it serves a second function—to produce the female hormones, estrogen and progesterone.

It doesn't seem possible that only three hundred years ago sperm were completely unknown. After sperm were discovered, there arose two opposing schools of thought. One group maintained that sperm originate life; the other that the egg is responsible. Astonishingly, for the next hundred years no one thought of the answer—that it required the marriage of the two.

Sperm are produced by the testicles. The word testicle has the same Latin derivation as testimony and testify and means "little witness." (In Biblical times it was apparently the custom for a man to swear an oath by his testicles, holding them with his hand.) An average ejaculation, amounting to a teaspoon of fluid, contains as many as five hundred million sperm.

The sperm cell, which contributes the husband's portion of hereditary material at fertilization, originates in threadlike tubes in the testicles. Like the ova of the mother, the sperm cells of the father begin to mature at puberty. Unlike the mother, however, whose egg-cell production ceases at menopause, the father continues to produce sperm cells throughout his life.

A mature spermatozoon (sperm for short) is very much smaller than an ovum. So tiny are they that all the sperm needed to repopulate the entire world could be fitted into a single raindrop. The spermatozoon measures only 1/6000 of an inch in diameter and is 1/500 of an inch in length; that is, the tail of a sperm is about twelve times the length or width of the head.

Under the microscope sperm look like little tadpoles, each with a tail that moves very fast and propels the sperm across the microscopic field. It is always a dramatic sight.

During sexual intercourse, sperm are forcefully ejected toward the cervix, the entrance into the womb. An initial wave of one hundred to two hundred million sperm reaches this port of entry and attempts to secure a beachhead. Whether these sperm find a friendly or a hostile reception depends upon the nature of the cervical secretions at that time. For several days near the time of ovulation, the normally dense, impenetrable cervical mucus becomes clear, favoring sperm entry and conception.

With favorable conditions, many sperm from the initial wave do gain immediate entry. Microscopic examination of samples of cervical secretion of women within *minutes* after intercourse have shown this to be the case. In fact, the cervical secretions will continue to show large numbers of motile sperm for many hours after intercourse, the basis for the so-called post-coital or after-intercourse test which is discussed in Chapter 7.

The majority of the millions of sperm ejaculated fail to gain entry into the cervix and are killed off by the normally hostile vaginal secretions. However, those that have passed into the cervix are no longer subject to vaginal secretions. Instead, they are well protected by the normally favorable cervical secretions (at mid-cycle at least). In that comfortable environment they can linger while preparing for the much longer journey to come.

This fantastic journey is as exciting as any tale in mythology—and what odds! Of the five hundred million sperm originally ejaculated, only a few dozen make the last lap of the journey leading directly to the egg itself, and of these only a few are destined actually to penetrate the ovum, with only one actually fertilizing the egg. It is the first microscopic act of sexual congress.

When this spermatozoon contacts the surface of the ovum, its activity stops; all is quiet. If enough time has passed, a complex process, known as capacitation, enhances the fertilizing potential of the sperm. Finally the head of the sperm enters the ovum and the tail separates, like a space capsule, eventually disappearing. The sperm is then drawn toward the center of the ovum. It carries the father's threads of inheritance (chromosomes), which will now merge with the mother's chromosomes. These chromosomes contain thousands of small units called genes, specifying the genetic inherited characteristics of new life. Whether the child will be a boy or a girl is determined solely by the sperm, which also carries the sex-determining chromosome.

Actually, in order to be fertilized, an egg must encounter a sperm within about two days, at which time the egg will still be near the outer end of the fallopian tube. Sperm cells, however, have a much longer life span than an ovum. They remain alive and motile for several days, and may be capable of fertilizing for much of that time. Nor do they have to arrive exactly at the time of ovulation. They can arrive several days before it, or shortly after it—which means that *there are about four or five days in each monthly cycle during which pregnancy can take place*.

Since only one sperm can fertilize (out of perhaps a half billion in a single ejaculation), it means that you had only a one-in-five-hundred-million chance to be you! If it had been any other of those five hundred million that had fertilized your mother's ovum, you would have been an entirely different person (and note how different siblings are), maybe even of the opposite sex.

When the ovum is fertilized by the sperm, the first step is the merging of their nuclei. The ovum then begins a series of cell divisions while still in the outer end of the tube. The egg itself does not increase in bulk at this time but simply divides into two, then four, then eight—and so on—smaller cells. Soon the fertilized ovum begins to look like a tiny mulberry, and each of the smaller cells within the ovum has a complete set of forty-six chromosomes, half from the father's sperm and half from the original unfertilized ovum. These forty-six chromosomes will be reproduced in each of the nuclei of the countless millions of body cells of the new individual.

It takes about four to five days for the tiny cluster to drift down the tube into the uterus. By the end of a week it has usually come to rest in one spot in the womb, whose lining is now well prepared. In this area it will take root, a process known as implantation or nesting. A few blood vessels may be broken during this phase, sometimes resulting in harmless "implantation staining."

SEX AND THE BIOLOGY OF REPRODUCTION

As early as the twelfth to the fourteenth day after conception, the tiny cluster of cells begins to form an embryo. It is about this time that menstruation would ordinarily have occurred. But no period comes. The woman is pregnant.

26

PREGNANCY TESTS

A woman hoping to conceive after years of barren marriage is very conscious of pregnancy tests. She is understandably impatient, and will want to know as soon as possible if pregnancy exists.

EARLY SIGNS OF PREGNANCY

If she has been keeping a temperature graph, it will give the earliest positive sign, based on the number of days of temperature elevation. She can then suspect pregnancy when only two or three days overdue, and be quite certain when four days overdue.

The most important method of detecting pregnancy is actually the pelvic examination, which should disclose a softening of the uterus and, in time, a gradual enlarging. But *early* detection of pregnancy by pelvic examination is difficult, as softening of the womb also occurs, for example, premenstrually. A slightly enlarged womb is significant, but only if the doctor can compare its size to previous examination, since not all non-pregnant uteri are the same size.

GENERAL SYMPTOMS

Then, of course, there are the various collateral symptoms. "Morning sickness" is the term commonly used to describe the nausea that troubles about 50 percent of pregnant women. Although it usually starts when a woman is about two weeks late, it may occur even earlier. Other early signs of pregnancy are swelling of the breasts, a feeling of bloating, and fatigue.

PREGNANCY TESTS

Whenever there are favorable signs and symptoms, most women prefer the additional assurance of a formal pregnancy test.

Pregnancy tests are based on the detection of a specific hormone, human chorionic gonadotropin (HCG). This hormone is produced by the placenta, the structure that nourishes the embryo (the placenta is known as the afterbirth after delivery). The amount of HCG produced by the embryonic placenta is often enough for detection as early as four to five days before a missed period in some of the more sensitive tests, and by ten to fourteen days in less sensitive ones. However, if a woman is already two or three weeks "late," almost any pregnancy test will have increased accuracy.

THE A-Z TEST

Now obsolete, this test involved the injection of a small quantity of the woman's urine into a test animal. The first such test was developed in 1928 by Drs. Aschheim and Zondek and is still known by their initials as the "A-Z" test. A small amount of the woman's urine is injected into a female mouse. If the woman is pregnant the HCG hormone in her urine will cause changes in the animal's ovaries within about forty-eight hours.

THE "RABBIT TEST"

A "rabbit test" is simply a modified version of the A-Z test, using that animal instead of a mouse. Another variation utilizes frogs, and gives results within several hours; either the woman's urine or her blood serum may be used.

IMMUNOLOGICAL REACTION TESTS

Newer methods, not requiring any animals, depend upon an immunological reaction similar to blood typing. They have the advantage of taking a much shorter time—from one minute to a few hours. In general, in early pregnancy "quickie" tests are less accurate than those taking several hours.

RADIORECEPTOR ASSAY

An important breakthrough in the field of testing for pregnancy was the development of the radioreceptor assay (RRA), blood test which is so sensitive that it is capable of detecting minute amounts of the pregnancy hormone (human chorionic gonadotropin; HCG) even several days *before* a missed period. It has particularly valuable application in questionable miscarriage and tubal pregnancy.

FALSE PREGNANCY

In some cases, women who are severely frustrated by their inability to conceive may experience a "psychological pregnancy," including all the typical symptoms that go with it—late period, "morning sickness," swelling of the breasts, etc. However, in these cases the pregnancy test is negative, and examination discloses no enlargement of the womb. This is a situation in which the subconscious is playing tricks, and it requires the most compassionate tact and reassurance.

GLOSSARY

Abortion: The premature termination of early pregnancy.

Adrenal: A gland of internal secretion, located near each kidney.

Amenorrhea: The absence of menstrual periods.

Anemia: A condition in which the red corpuscles of the blood are reduced in number, or are deficient in hemoglobin.

Basal body temperature: Temperature readings taken immediately upon awakening.

Biopsy: A snip of tissue taken for detailed examination.

Caesarean section: Surgical removal of a baby from the uterus.

Capacitation: The process by which spermatozoa become able to penetrate the egg surface.

Chromosomes: Threads of inheritance, present in nuclei of all cells.

Chronic: Lasting a long time.

Clomiphene: A synthetic non-hormonal chemical, commonly used to stimulate ovulation.

Coitus: Sexual intercourse.

Corpus luteum: The area from which the egg was extruded from the ovary.

Culdoscopy: An operative procedure in which an instrument is placed through the vagina to visualize the pelvic organs.

Diagnosis: The doctor's identification of a particular disease or abnormality.

Donor insemination: Artificial insemination of a woman using sperm other than her husband's.

Ectopic pregnancy: A pregnancy located outside the womb, usually in the tube.

Embryo: An organism in the early stages of its development.

Endocrine glands: Glands that produce hormones that pass directly into the blood stream and affect body functions.

Endometriosis: The presence of bits of uterine lining outside the womb, a disorder often associated with infertility.

Endometrium: The inner lining of the womb.

Endoscopy: An operative procedure in which an instrument is placed either through the abdomen (laparoscopy) or through the vagina (culdoscopy) to visualize the pelvic organs.

Estrogen: The chief female sex hormone, produced mainly in the ovary.

Fallopian tubes: The oviducts; tubes which transport the egg from the womb.

Fibroids: Fibro-muscular benign growths arising in the wall of the womb.

Frigidity: Female sexual indifference or "coldness."

FSH: Follicle-stimulating hormone from the pituitary gland, which stimulates the growth of ovarian egg follicles.

Habitual abortion: At least three consecutive miscarriages.

Hymen: The membrane covering the entrance to the vagina.

Hypothalamus: The midbrain, sometimes called the seat of the emotions.

Hysterosalpingography: An x-ray of the lining of the uterus and tubes.

Impotence: Inability of the male to carry out sexual intercourse or to ejaculate.

Incompetent cervix: A weakness of the neck of the womb, believed to be responsible for some cases of late miscarriage around the fifth or sixth month.

Infertility: The inability to conceive.

Insufflation of the tubes: The passage of carbon dioxide gas through the tubes; the Rubin test.

Laparoscopy: An operative procedure in which an instrument is placed through the abdomen to visualize the pelvic organs.

LH: Luteinizing hormone from the pituitary gland, which triggers ovulation.

Menopause: The permanent end of menstruation and fertility.

Ovulation: The release of an egg (ovum) by the ovary.

Pergonal: An extract of pituitary hormone used to stimulate ovulation, often associated with multiple births.

Pituitary: An important gland located at the base of the brain.

Placenta: The structure attached to the womb that nourishes the embryo or fetus; the afterbirth.

Post-coital test: An examination of the cervical secretions after intercourse.

Progesterone: A female sex hormone produced by the corpus luteum after ovulation to prepare the lining of the womb for implantation of the fertilized egg.

Retroversion: Tipped backward, as applied to the position of the womb.

Rubin test: The passage of carbon dioxide gas through the tubes (tubal insufflation).

Salpingitis: Inflammation of the tubes.

Salpingo-hysterography: X-ray of the tubes and uterus.

Semen: The total fluid ejaculate of the male, containing the sperm.

Stein-Leventhal Syndrome: Polycystic ovaries often associated with infertility.

Sterility: Infertility.

"Test-Tube Baby": A term that has been varyingly applied to (1) artificial insemination with donor sperm (AID); (2) artificial insemination with husband sperm (AIH); and (3), most popularly, to fertilization in vitro (outside the body) with reimplantation into the womb.

Vaginismus: Involuntary contractions of the muscles surrounding the vagina.

Varicocele: Varicose veins in the male scrotum, sometimes associated with lessened fertility.

Venereal disease: Diseases contracted by sexual intercourse, such as gonorrhea and syphilis.

INDEX

A

Abortion, 15, 27, 30, 90–91, 167, 169
  defined, 197
  habitual, 90, 97–98, 118
  illegal, 19
  induced, 19
  missed, 90, 99
  "silent," 66
  spontaneous, *see*
    Miscarriage
Abstinence, 109
Adhesions, pelvic, 78, 81
  intrauterine, 118
  postoperative, 85
Adoption, 132–48
  of foreign children, 136, 138–39 (*list*), 147–48 (*list*)
  information sources, 147–48
  physician's role in, 134
  problems and prospects in, 134–36
  sources, 136–48 (*list*)
Adrenals, 45, 186
  defined, 197
After-intercourse test, *see*
  Post-coital test

Age and fertility, 9–11
Allergy to sperm as cause of infertility, 116–17
Amenorrhea, 71–72
  defined, 197
American Fertility Society, 25
American Medical Association, 165
Amniocentesis, 175
Anatomy, 11–18
  infertility caused by anatomical factors, 12–14
  sex, 40–41, 179–81
Anemia, defined, 197
Artificial insemination, 109–10, 172
  erectile impotence and, 49
  husband insemination, 46–47, 56
  intrauterine, 56, 164
  by partitioned ejaculate, 46–47
  semen banks, 130
  test-tube births and, 164–65
  See also Donor insemination; Test-tube births
A-Z test, 194–95

Prostate gland, 41
Prostitutes, infertility of, 117
Psychological infertility, 16–18, 31, 83–84
  adoption and, 148–49
  emotional factors, 16, 18, 87–89
  of men, 48–50

R

"Rabbit test," 195
Radioreceptor assay (RRA), 101, 195
Reappraisal of infertility, 115–75
  parenthood in spite of infertility, see Donor insemination; Test-tube births
  by testing, 116–17
Religious view
  of donor insemination, 125
  of test-tube births, 160, 165
Reproductive process, 187–92; see also Conception; Intercourse; Menstruation; Pregnancies
Retroversion, 13, 97
  defined, 199
Rh blood factor, 98, 128
Rock, Dr. John, 152–53
Rubin (gas insufflation) test, 35, 78–80, 81, 83, 103
  defined, 199

S

Salpingitis, defined, 199
Salpingo-hysterography, 80–81
  defined, 199

Scrotum, 40, 46, 51
Secondary (one-child) infertility, 102–5
Semen, defined, 199; see Sperm
Seminal vesicles, 41
Sex anatomy, 40–41, 179–81
Sex life and infertility, see Marital life
Shettles, Dr. Landrum, 172
  Choose Your Baby's Sex, 173
Sims, Dr. James Marion, 5–6, 53, 54
Sims-Huhner test, 53–55
Soranus, 4–5
Specialists, consultation *re* infertility, 25–27
Speculum, vaginal, 6
Sorenson decision *re* donor insemination, 124
Specialists consulted about infertility, 25
Sperm (spermatozoa, semen), 5, 24, 34, 40–48
  allergy as cause of infertility, 116–17
  count, 43–44, 46
  deficiency of, 45, 47
  flow from vagina, 12
  frozen, 47
  function, 188–91
  lack of, 48
  life, 55
  migration, 53–54
  morphology, 45
  motility of, 11, 43–45, 46, 51
  normal, 41–42
  production of, 40–41, 188–89
  weak, 46–47, 55, 107
  X (girl) and Y (boy), 174–75

ABOUT THE AUTHOR

DR. SHERWIN A. KAUFMAN is an Associate Attending in Obstetrics and Gynecology at Lenox Hill Hospital, New York City, and is director of its Infertility Clinic. In private practice for thirty years, he is a member of the American Fertility Society and a Fellow of the American College of Obstetricians and Gynecologists and the American College of Surgeons. He is medical consultant to Planned Parenthood of New York City, having served as medical director for over twenty years. Dr. Kaufman has co-authored two medical texts, *Infertility in Women* and *Modern Office Gynecology* and has published extensively in professional journals. He has written several books for the general public, including *The Ageless Woman*, which deals with menopause and the middle years, and *From A Gynecologist's Notebook: Questions Women Ask,* which provides answers to the most common queries in his field. He lives in Manhattan with his wife and the youngest of three sons. He enjoys golf, tennis, writing and is an accomplished pianist.

Congratulations—But...

what about all those questions and problems that arrive with a new addition to the family? Here are several invaluable books for any new or expectant mother. They are filled with helpful hints for raising healthy children in a happy home. Best of luck and may all your problems be little ones!

☐	13742	**BETTER HOMES AND GARDENS BABY BOOK**	$2.50
☐	13085	**UNDERSTANDING PREGNANCY AND CHILDBIRTH** by Sheldon H. Cherry, M.D.	$2.25
☐	12359	**PREGNANCY NOTEBOOK** by Marcia Morton	$1.95
☐	13246	**NINE MONTHS READING** by Robert E. Hall, M.D.	$2.25
☐	12640	**FEED ME! I'M YOURS** by Vicki Lansky	$2.25
☐	12216	**SIX PRACTICAL LESSONS FOR AN EASIER CHILDBIRTH** by Elisabeth Bing	$2.25
☐	10409	**CHILDBIRTH AT HOME** by Marion Sousa	$1.95
☐	13624	**NAME YOUR BABY** by Lareina Rule	$2.25
☐	12335	**YOUR BABY'S SEX: NOW YOU CAN CHOOSE** by Rorvik & Shettles, M.D.'s	$1.95
☐	13901	**THE FIRST TWELVE MONTHS OF LIFE** by Frank Caplan, ed.	$2.95
☐	13182	**COMPLETE BOOK OF BREASTFEEDING** by M. Eiger, M.D. & S. Olds	$2.25
☐	13711	**IMMACULATE DECEPTION** by Suzanne Arms	$2.95
☐	12844	**PREPARING FOR PARENTHOOD** by Lee Salk	$2.25
☐	12497	**PREGNANCY: THE PSYCHOLOGICAL EXPERIENCE** by Arthur & Libby Colman	$2.25
☐	13699	**MAKING YOUR OWN BABY FOOD** by James Turner	$1.95
☐	13961	**MOVING THROUGH PREGNANCY** by Elisabeth Bing	$2.25
☐	01271	**MAKING LOVE DURING PREGNANCY** Bing & Colman	$6.95

Buy them at your local bookstore or use this handy coupon for ordering: